MW01094141

Fixing the Aftermath of Having Kids, No Matter How Long Ago It Was

WTF HAPPENED TO MY BODY?

NATALIE
GARAY

Copyright © 2025 by Natalie Garay

All rights reserved. No part of this book may be reproduced,
stored in a retrieval system or transmitted, in any form
or by any means, without the prior written consent of the
publisher, except in the case of brief quotations,
embodied in reviews and articles.

First things first, I am not your doctor so do us both
a favor and check in with yours first before beginning any
exercise practice. This book is not intended as a substitute
for the medical advice of physicians. The reader should
regularly consult a physician in matters relating to
his/her/their health and particularly with respect to any
symptoms that may require diagnosis or medical attention.

Cataloguing in publication information
is available from Library and Archives Canada.
ISBN 978-1-77458-542-9 (paperback)
ISBN 978-1-77458-543-6 (ebook)

Page Two
pagetwo.com

Edited by Sarah Brohman
Copyedited by Merlina McGovern
Proofread by Alison Strobel
Cover and interior design by Taysia Louie
Interior illustrations by Michelle Clement

nataliesayswtf.com

To my nuggets—Nia, Kaia, and Ava

CONTENTS

IT'S NEVER TOO LATE
TO REHABILITATE

N THE FALL OF 1999, I made a huge solo move to Los Angeles. I was starry-eyed, full of wonder, and brimming over with naivete. I was ready to dance my way onto all the stages and big screens. I had just graduated from the University of California, Santa Barbara, with my bachelor's degree in dance, an excellent program that I auditioned for on a whim. I didn't know what I wanted to do in life, but I knew that attempting to study anything else would just bore me to tears, and, frankly, I didn't have the mental focus to sit in a classroom all day, every day.

After a couple of years of glamorous cattle-call dance auditions (I bombed horribly at an audition for a Britney Spears video), many dance classes, some acting classes (because I "couldn't just be a dancer," according to my agents), and waiting tables at California Pizza Kitchen, I discovered that I was pregnant. At that time, it wasn't the best news, so I tried to deny the reality of it at first. I was just getting started in my dance career, and my relationship, if you could even call it that, with the father was new. I was twenty-six years old at the time. Not extremely young, but young enough to know that I was not ready for a child in any capacity.

Even though the universe kept showing me signs that I was pregnant everywhere I went, I delayed finding out for sure. Despite being scared sh*tless, I finally made an appointment to see a doctor—who confirmed what I was afraid of: I was definitely pregnant. Not long after my initial appointment, I was scheduled for an ultrasound to make sure everything looked normal, but normal was not in the cards for my case. The ultrasound showed me that, sure enough, I was pregnant—not with one baby, but two. Holy sh*t!

This was definitely not in the plans. Not in *my* plans anyway. Apparently, the universe had another idea for me. Little did I know at the time that motherhood was going to be the ultimate journey, life lesson, and growth process I could possibly experience. But I wasn't going to learn about it with just one baby. Nope, I had to go big and grow two babies. This was a life lesson on steroids. And, according to my grandmother, when I do something, I *really* do it (thanks, GG). Go big or go home, eh?

I continued to dance while still somewhat in denial that I was pregnant, or maybe it was shock. I attended ballet classes, performed in some small shows, and pretended that my growing belly and I weren't taking up any extra space. I kept this up until my seventh month, at which point, my dance career came to a screeching halt. I knew that continuing to dance wasn't going to hurt the babies, but my body wanted me to slow down.

My pregnancy was considered high risk because, you know, I was growing two humans. That meant multiple ultrasounds to make sure things continued to stay on track. Twins typically do arrive earlier than their due date, but I felt great throughout my pregnancy. I enjoyed being pregnant, well, once I got over that initial shock.

After yet another routine ultrasound, the doctor looked concerned. "Are you feeling that?" she asked. "No," I replied, not knowing what she was talking about. Then she said, "You're having contractions. It's too early for you to have contractions. If they continue, you could deliver too early."

This was in early September, but my due date wasn't until mid-December. And even if twins do tend to come early, it was far too early for them to be delivered. The doctor made the call to admit me to the hospital to keep these babies in and cooking for as long as possible. I was given magnesium to stop the contractions (which made me feel like sh*t), and the babies were given something to help their lungs grow more quickly in case they arrived too early.

The hospital became my new home. Bedridden, I was only allowed out of bed for bathroom visits. I refused to use the bedpan since I couldn't even lift my ass over it. Weeks went by. Boredom set in. I watched the MLB World Series at night and tried to read during the day between visits with family and friends. Thank goodness for those visits. The nurses became my friends, and they took incredible care of me, washing my hair as I hung my head over the foot of my bed and toasting my crappy hospital bagel—all the little things that made the experience as good as it could be, I suppose.

Many long and scary nights went by, and, after two months of holding the twins in for as long as I could, they decided to make their debut a full month before their due date. No amount of magnesium was going to stop my contractions this time. And since the babies were still so small, I needed to have a C-section—this was go-time.

Up until now, I'd never had a major surgery or even had to stay in bed for a long period. Both did a huge number on my body. I've always been active, from playing youth soccer throughout high school to participating on the swimming team and playing water polo to all that time I spent dancing. Lying in bed was the hardest thing for me to do. But worse, after being bedbound for two months and going through major abdominal surgery, my body was wrecked! My muscles had atrophied so much that I couldn't even walk. How was I expected to care for my babies if my body wasn't even functioning properly?

But these little nuggets were coming whether I was ready or not, and man were they tiny. They arrived on November 11, 2002, Veterans Day, one weighing in at a whopping five pounds, nine ounces, and the other at three pounds, eleven ounces. (My mom suggested naming them Freedom and Liberty. Yikes.) At that point, I was struggling to relearn how to sit up in bed, get out of bed, and sit in a chair. I was also learning how to pump and feed two babies, who weren't even in the room with me but in the NICU on another floor. The bed and chair ordeal happened multiple times a day just so I could get up to see and try to feed them. And I only had five days to figure this all out before I was kicked out of the hospital. After two months, I was ready to get the f*ck out of the hospital, but after my C-section, I wasn't so sure how I was going to manage it all.

When I was released, twin A, my little Nia, came with me. She had passed the weight requirement for release and was breathing well on her own. Twin B, Kaia, was still itty-bitty. Because she weighed in at less than four pounds, she had to stay in the NICU longer until she could put on a few more pounds. I returned to the hospital daily to hold and feed my little peanut, Kaia. She had an incredible team around her who cheered her on every day. The nurses commented on how tiny, but mighty, she was (she was a fighter, and, twenty-plus years later, she still is). It took some juggling so I could spend time with Kaia. My mom and dad, or sometimes the twins' dad (he's a long, dramatic, and dumb story), would sit with Nia outside of the NICU since she wasn't allowed back in.

Two weeks later, the day before Thanksgiving, we broke Kaia out of NICU jail. She had gained enough weight, so the doctors cleared her to go home. We loaded up the car and headed home straight to my parents' house three hours away. We ended up staying through the holidays so that my parents could help me with the twins. What a f*cking whirlwind.

My time in the hospital had passed excruciatingly slowly, and it took a toll on my physical and mental health. Initially, the doctors had told me that the twins would need to stay in the hospital for a month, maybe longer, because they had arrived early and were so small. Thankfully, that wasn't the case, but I was extremely nervous to take them home. At least I knew they were safe in the hospital. If something was wrong, an alarm on their machines would immediately sound. One kind nurse felt the need to remind me that I wouldn't have these machines at home. That didn't ease my worries at all. On top of that, I had this scar across my belly and a weak body. When I left the hospital, the only information or instructions I received were not to drive too soon, not to pick up anything heavy, and to walk a little. That's it. Everything else I had to learn on my own.

The small amount of information the doctor did give me struck me as odd. I didn't get why I shouldn't drive until I did exactly that. I needed to run a simple errand, but while I was on my way home, I suddenly had to hit the brakes in the car. That action activated my newly severed abdominals, and holy sh*t did it hurt. At that exact moment, I remembered the doctor's words. Guess I should have listened to the little information that he did give me.

I am baffled by the totally inadequate information the health system gives to moms about how to support their bodies after pregnancy and birth when they leave the hospital. Instead, women find themselves playing a f*cking guessing game. And forget about any mental support you might need for the roller coaster of emotions you'll go through as your body readjusts to a postpartum world. The world still dismisses those feelings as the baby blues or postpartum depression, shrugging them off as "part of the territory" of pregnancy and delivery. The image that comes to my mind when a mom is released from the hospital is the doctor quickly waving her off and saying, "Off you go now. Good luck!" in a "Don't let the door hit you on the ass" sort of way.

Unless you are surrounded by a supportive community of moms who are open and willing to share their experiences and unless you read obsessively about pregnancy and postpartum issues, you may find yourself unprepared for life after birth. Instead, you end up fumbling your way through this fragile and important time in your life and learning from your mistakes. It's hard not to feel miserable when you are failing every single day.

Here's the good news. I've done the fumbling for you, and I'm willing to share my results. I'm going to share what I've learned through not only my own experience, but also while helping other women to heal. I'll also share some client stories from my two decades of teaching Pilates, in studio and online, and helping women rehabilitate from the effects of pregnancy and birth. All that experience has come together in what I call the Natalie Garay Methode.

The Natalie Garay Methode

The Natalie Garay Methode recognizes that there's more to us than just skin, bones, and muscles. I developed this method inspired by my experience dealing with and healing my own sh*t. From my bed-rest ordeal to being a solo mama in survival mode, I was on a hunt to find ways to not lose my f*cking sanity. Based on my own experience and that of my clients over the years, I've created a method that combines the movement practice and principles of Pilates, an understanding of your energy through the ancient Indian system of the chakras, and flower essence therapy.

The Natalie Garay Methode is tailored to all mothers who need to rehabilitate after vaginal or C-section deliveries. I'm going to explain why you don't just need to rehabilitate your physical body after pregnancy and delivery; you also need to be curious and aware of your emotional and energetic bodies. You may be thinking, "WTF are those?" Don't worry; I will talk about these later in the book.

As you read this book, you'll quickly realize that the core of my rehabilitation method is Pilates. I was introduced to Pilates while I was pregnant with my twins, but I didn't truly realize the benefits until after my bed-rest stint. Soon after I had my third daughter, I decided to become certified as a Pilates instructor with Core Conditioning Physical Therapy in Sherman Oaks, California. A few years later, I was certified as a Master Pilates instructor with Pilates Sports Center (PSC) in Encino, California, to further hone my skills and get more in-depth training. I have also trained as a flower essence therapist, and I use this modality in my method.

Over the past twenty years, I've taught workshops at various studios as well as at my own studio, online and in person. I've created video libraries and online courses, and I've been a guest lecturer and speaker for various mom groups at studios, hospitals, and childbirth support groups. I also taught Pilates in physical therapy clinics, working alongside doctors of physical therapy (DPTs) and assisting

Feeling sh*tty is not a life sentence.

in their patients' postoperative care. I love sharing what I've learned so that moms don't have to fumble along in pain and hopelessness.

When my ability to move and dance freely changed suddenly, it was really f*cking scary, and I was full of questions. As I moved and healed my own body, I learned more about the parts of the body that we often ignore but that play a huge role in our daily quality of life. The more you understand that it's important to take the time to listen to your body, the better you will feel. And that knowledge will help you in the long run when it comes to mothering and life. I'm going to walk you through how I healed my body after spending two months on bed rest, followed by a C-section, while also trying not to lose it as I did all of this completely solo. (Yup, as I said, a total sh*t show.)

This book is the guide you need after having kids, no matter how long ago it was.

Read that again: *no matter how long ago it was*.

After twenty-plus years of being a mother and two decades of working with moms, I've discovered that when the body starts talking through pain, aches, and lethargy, we don't connect these symptoms to the birth of our children from years before. When we do make that connection, we can get to the root cause of the problems and rebuild what changed and shifted as we created a whole f*cking human with our body.

Mothers should not have to suffer through life after bringing a child into the world. Just the opposite. We should be doing everything we can to support them and help them feel their best and to heal properly. So that's why

I am sounding the alarm with this book. If only we were supported like the MF-ing badasses that we are for creating life and given the tools we require after having kids, we would be that much more powerful.

Are you feeling me?

This is the guidebook that you should have received when you left the hospital. The owner's manual to putting your bits back together and to feeling like yourself again. Yes, becoming a mother is a major life transition, a welcome one. But you shouldn't have to limp through it when, with just a few simple tools and some vital information, you can easily thrive. Read this book with curiosity and ask yourself what you could use and benefit from. Discuss it with other moms in your life because it's never too late to get support for what you need to help you feel like yourself again.

How to Use This Book

Since you've picked up this book, I'm going to assume that you also have an affinity for using the word f*ck and that you don't want a sh*t life. I specialize in helping clients recover and rehabilitate from C-sections, diastasis recti, and a weakened pelvic floor. While some of the information I have about those issues might not apply to you, the information about rehabilitation and healing after pregnancy and the accompanying exercises and tools I have gathered together in part three are relevant because all mamas need to rehab their abs after pregnancy.

Now that we've gotten those background items out of the way, you'll see that I've organized this book into three parts.

In the first part, I will talk about your physical body and what happens during pregnancy, birth, and a C-section surgery, as well as how to fix the aftermath. This book starts with a look at your physical body because this is your foundation. How strong your body is determines how well you can stand, walk, and move around. After my C-section, I discovered just how important abdominal strength is for helping me get up and down out of chairs. This is the largest section of the book because, hey, it's your body, the container you are walking around in. Moving your body is the easiest way to move energy and release anything that's stored and isn't necessary for you to hold on to anymore. Movement is the best medicine and therapy for all bodies but especially after birth or C-section surgery.

In the second part of the book, I will talk about other parts of you that you need to address after you've had kids, but that you might be less familiar with: your energetic and emotional bodies. The information I share in this part of the book is as important as the symptoms you may experience during and after pregnancy in your physical body. That's because symptoms of problems in the emotional and energetic bodies can be subtle and difficult to pin down, which means they have the potential to be even more debilitating.

In part two, I'll also share some stories that have inspired me to look more deeply at how the body functions. Through my yoga practice and learning about the ancient

Indian system of energy centers called the chakras, I understood why I felt so much joy and relief through movement. I have also learned to help myself and my clients release stagnant energy through flower essence therapy—sweet, gentle remedies that can be life-changing for mamas who are seeking to feel more grounded and gain back some ease in their lives.

Finally, in part three, I'll give you some tools, practices, and exercises that will help you feel like yourself again! You've heard me say it before—and I'll keep saying it—it doesn't matter how long ago you had your kids, you can still benefit greatly from rehabilitation.

When you are limited by a lack of strength, your ability to perform simple daily activities will take a toll on you mentally and emotionally. You will feel the limitations of your body, and it will cause you to feel a range of emotions from anger to frustration and even hopelessness, which can drastically change the quality of your life. Keeping up with my physical and mental wellness practices is incredibly important to me because these practices allow me to live each day fully. I want to feel energized, clear-minded, and happy. I want optimal health and well-being as much as possible. That doesn't mean I feel amazing every single day. But I feel great more times than not, and when I'm not feeling great, I have tools to support me.

I want this for everyone, but especially for moms. I want you to be able to feel strong inside and out. When you do, you'll feel more confident, more energized, and have an increased will to take care of your toddlers, teenagers, and young adults. But this health and well-being won't come by itself; it takes some work. And you're going to need all the help you can get with all of it, my friend. This book will stimulate your curiosity about what's going on with your body and show you how to fix what's been nagging at you and taking away from your daily life. Now is the time for you to get moving toward your healthy life, no matter how long ago you were pregnant.

Are you f*cking ready?

YOUR FOUNDATION: YOUR PHYSICAL BODY

1

ARE YOU F*CKING LISTENING?

A FEW DAYS AFTER I was released from my hospital stint, my C-section incision started to feel heavy and looked odd. I didn't know what it was or why this was happening, but I knew it couldn't be normal. Rather than ignore it and hope that the feeling would pass, I went back to the hospital to have it looked at. After having lived there for two months, I felt comfortable going right up to "my floor" and asking my nurse buddies to have a look. (Did I mention that I even had my baby shower there? Right in the doctors' lounge.)

At first sight, the nurses could see that something was off—the incision was red and didn't appear to be healing properly. One of the nurses took a stick of some sort and poked at it to release some fluid that had collected under my stapled incision. Gross! Even though the skin around my incision was still numb, I could feel the fluid drain over my stomach and down onto the table. What I learned was that this could happen on occasion after a C-section. I was prescribed antibiotics and instructed to clean and repack my incision with gauze every couple of days until the incision closed fully, which could take a few weeks. As if using the bathroom after a C-section wasn't hard enough; I now had to perform a minor procedure on my incision every few days. I had no idea that this could happen.

I could have easily dismissed this "odd" feeling. I could have easily ignored it, especially because I had so much going on. At the time, I was caring for Nia, who was at home, but also making daily visits to the hospital to visit Kaia in the NICU. But I *knew* something was off. I could feel it, and I needed to take care of it. I listened to my body. I listened to my intuition telling me that something was off. Who knows what might have happened if I hadn't gone back to the hospital? Maybe nothing. Maybe everything. A minor infected incision might have turned into a major infection, which could have led to another surgery or who knows what. And that would have made my healing process longer and my days even more challenging. Nobody needs that.

We have all ignored a symptom at one time or another—an achy shoulder or back, a ringing in the ear, or ongoing fatigue. We brush things off as a symptom of aging or exhaustion. Or maybe we've been conditioned to ignore it, suck it up, and wear our ailments like a badge of honor. WTF?

I'm guessing that you don't want to call it a day at three in the afternoon from exhaustion or skip adventures for fear of pissing your pants. And you're definitely not ready to settle into a rocking chair at age fifty, right? I'm north of forty, and I'm just getting started. I want to have a healthy lifestyle because I want to be full of energy. I want to have clear focus and optimal strength to live fully every single day so that I can do whatever I want without restriction.

If you're like me, you want to live your life fully without limitation. You want to do anything and everything to make sure that you have all the energy, focus, and mind clarity to enjoy your life while you can. What if, instead of ignoring these simple messages from your body, you paused, got curious, and asked yourself what this could be—what is your body trying to tell you?

Now is the time to investigate. What do you need to help you feel better right now? Do you have a list of tools or go-to remedies? Ask yourself questions. Find out what you need and what may have caused your current state or condition. And then, don't ignore it—f*cking fix it!

Taking Care of Yourself Is an Active Decision

Not dealing with your physical symptoms can really f*ck up the rest of your life. Overriding or ignoring your physical needs—or any needs, for that matter—leaves you significantly deficient and incapable of fulfilling anything else, from simple daily tasks to doing the things you really enjoy.

Your quality of life depends on how you care for your body. So, it's up to you to make the best decisions possible to care for it. Nobody can do that for you. Nobody can force you to move your body, to eat well, or to get enough sleep. These are all choices that you need to make. Ignoring your body can lead to injury or just feeling pissed and burned out. This benefits nobody. It does nothing for you but stress you out, and for those around you, the results of ignoring those issues can be scary, to say the least. Nobody likes an unhappy mama.

I make the decision each day to do things that serve me well. Each morning, I tune in to my body and my energy to see what I need and how I'm feeling. This check-in guides my day. I will check to see what my energy level is, and this tells me if I have what it takes to have a highly productive day or if I need to take it easy. Even in the nonproductive moments, we're still quite productive, by the way.

My tune-in process starts with journaling, a brief meditation, and a routine in which I observe my body to see how it feels that day. After that, I move my body either with a walk; stretching; rebounding (jumping on a trampoline); or, my favorite activity, a few laps in the pool. For this astrological Cancer crab, the water is my healing place. If I still need a little more care after my movement practice, I take a bath.

You might be thinking, "How the f*ck am I supposed to fit all this into my day?" Well, it takes practice and time to incorporate what works best for you and your schedule. It took me some time to carve space for this regular check-in practice into my schedule, and now it's just something I do. But it's a choice. I make time for this tune-in, and I make it a habitual part of my day.

I'm not asking you to train for a marathon on day one. Whatever you choose to do can be as simple as a quick check-in with yourself. This will give you a feel for what you need to have the best day possible. Your body may be telling you that you are tired. This is a good day to give yourself grace and maybe skip a few things on your to-do list. We've all had sh*tty days that just get sh*ttier when we powered through them. If I'm not feeling good, what's the f*cking point? I'm so sick of this hustle culture and "no pain, no gain" bullsh*t. Not that you needed a permission slip, but here's your permission slip: it's okay to rest; it's okay to take things slow; and it's okay to NOT do something you don't feel like doing.

Rant over.

Training for Life

I recently decided to go back to school. I'm starting slowly by taking an introductory college algebra class because I haven't taken a math class in more than twenty years, and it's completely foreign to me. Reading the book and looking at the equations makes my head spin and my brain hurt. I've had to make some adjustments in my day to facilitate learning something new.

I need to fuel my body and my brain better, make sure I've had adequate sleep, and stay hydrated to stay focused, alert, and process this new foreign language. I know that taking care of my body and brain is crucial for being able to support my goals. Part of this care includes making time for thirty minutes of swimming a day as well. I look at this activity as if I'm training for life. I say that somewhat jokingly, but your daily habits will either help or hinder you in your life.

While training for life will look different for everyone, my point is that you need to take care of yourself, find what works for you, and determine why it matters to you. Finding your reason why is important; if you find your "why," it will become your driving force. You may want to just be able to keep up with your energetic kids. Maybe you want to work part-time or feel better throughout the day at your

Taking care of yourself is an active decision.

full-time job. You might even want to start a business of your own. Since my kids are now adults, I don't have to run after them, but I do need to have the mental clarity and sanity to help them navigate their transition into young adulthood. So, take some time to answer these four questions in your journal to find out what is driving you. Later, in part three, you will come back to review these goals.

1 What is it that you want to do in a day?
2 What do you want to accomplish in a month?
3 How about in five to ten years?
4 What will you need to be able to complete it?

You Are the Boss of Your Body

Did you get that?

You are the authority on your body and how you are feeling. Nobody knows you better than you do, even if you might not know your body very well—yet. But here's a scenario you might be familiar with.

You take the time to make an appointment to see your doctor because you're not feeling like yourself. You carve out the time to go to the appointment, arrange for the kids to be taken care of, or take the time off work. When you finally get to the doctor's office, you end up sitting in the waiting room watching prescription drug commercials so many times that you may ask your doctor if you're a candidate for one of them.

The nurse takes your vitals and checks you in, asking why you're here today, and you tell her. You break it down for her, all the symptoms, feelings, all the goods. Then you wait nervously for the doctor to race in, only to have to answer the same questions all over again. Why don't they communicate with each other?

Then here it comes, the response, "Oh that's normal, that's nothing to be worried about. You have three kids. Of course you're tired all the time. If things get worse, come back and see me." WTF? You slowly get dressed thinking to yourself what a f*cking waste of time that was. But you're also thinking that maybe he's right and you're crazy; maybe nothing is wrong with you. Maybe it *is* all in your head.

I've heard this story from moms so many times, and it infuriates me. We want support, we want answers, and we deserve to feel "normal." You know your body best, and you know when it's not functioning like you'd like it to. It's frustrating to be dismissed by your healthcare provider after making the decision and effort to seek help. But, like I said before, you know your body better than anyone else does.

Ask for what you want.

Do you need a specific test run? Ask for it. Need a referral to a specialist? Ask for it. Your doctor is not the authority on your body. Their input can be helpful, but don't let them have the final say. Working with a doctor or a healer of any kind should be a collaborative relationship, not one that feels one-sided and dismissive. If you don't get the answer or the support you want, find someone who will help you. You can seek more supportive care at any time. You do not need to stay with someone who doesn't listen to you or who doesn't do anything to help you.

Some go-to practitioners that I've found to be extremely supportive are my acupuncturist, chiropractor, hydrotherapist, massage therapist, and functional medicine doctor. All of them listen intently with care and compassion and always have great advice for treatments, things to avoid, or blood tests to run that might help us look deeper into a particular situation.

In my opinion, blood tests and brain scans will save us all. When my daughter and mother were experiencing their own health journeys, they both had brain scans and specific blood tests done. These gave us incredibly detailed pictures of what was happening with them. I eventually had these tests done as well for preventive health measures. This led to my obsession with functional medicine and prompted my decision to go back to school to become a naturopathic doctor. That's another story and another book. But if you are interested in more information on this subject, check out the videos of brain scans that Amen Clinics posts of its clientele. You can also learn more about functional medicine online or by following my go-to, Dr. Mark Hyman, founder and director of The UltraWellness Center.

Healing Is a Process of Investigation

Have you ever met a kid who just keeps asking, "Why?" You give them an answer, but they just keep asking, "But why?" That's me.

I want to know the "why." Why does someone have chronic pain? Why is someone acting like an asshole?

What's really going on? What's the root cause of this feeling or behavior? When you know the root cause of what is bothering you, then you can really take care of it and fix it—not just temporarily but permanently. I've never wanted a quick fix; I want to know what the deep-down cause is and start there.

There is always a reason. There is always a root cause. Like a sleuth, I will dig deep and ask the questions and go back as far as I can go to find the reason for why I am feeling a certain way. I like this approach so much more than masking feelings or symptoms. I don't want to patch up a bad feeling or take a pill. I want to know what's deficient, what needs support, and fill up accordingly.

The root cause of a problem is often different for every person—and so, too, is the solution. Each person needs their own personalized plan because one size does not fit all where your health is concerned.

As I mentioned earlier, when my daughter was experiencing a health crisis, we sought the help of a functional medicine doctor who ordered more than the standard blood work labs. Even before meeting with him, my daughter had to complete what seemed like four hundred f*cking pages of questions. The care he offered was so thorough.

What I loved about the blood work reports was that they gave the doctor the big picture of what was going on in my daughter's body. The results gave him a road map to support her. They showed him what her hormone levels were, which showed him what symptoms they were causing. The blood work also showed which nutrients and vitamins she was deficient in and what issues were resulting from those deficiencies. With this information, he knew which foods would support her body and which foods would increase inflammation or cause other reactions. It was brilliant. "Why isn't this standard? Everybody needs this." I thought this to myself, and said as much, many times, to the support staff, who agreed.

Rather than guessing which supplements to take, my daughter knew exactly what she needed to support her system and to help her obtain optimal body and brain function. It was incredible to see which symptoms were caused by a simple vitamin deficiency. If these tests could determine that a clinical deficiency of vitamin D or B was causing your depression, wouldn't you want to know that?

It works the same way for your physical body. When you know which muscles are weak and how to strengthen them to support and balance your body, the knowledge changes the game in the quality of your daily living. Wouldn't you want to know that your weakened butt muscles are causing your sciatica or back pain? With this knowledge, you could alleviate your symptoms with simple strengthening exercises. No more limping along through life unsure or practicing exercises that aren't effective.

2

IT'S ALL ABOUT THE ABS

T WASN'T until I signed up for a Pilates teacher training program in 2004 that I fully began to understand what a huge role our abdominals play in our daily functions. The abdominals support everything. They control how you sit, stand, lift, and walk, as well as hold things in place. Your pelvis is supported by your abdominals, butt muscles, inner thigh muscles, and, of course, your pelvic floor muscles. When these muscles are weak, your pelvis can become misaligned, causing your sciatic nerve to be pinched, which can then lead to pain shooting down the leg. Your pelvic alignment also affects your knees. If you have knee pain, strengthen that butt and those abs.

Learning how all of these issues were connected to our abdominals opened my eyes to how major a C-section surgery is. I experienced this surgery twice, but it wasn't until I learned what the abdominals are responsible for that the seriousness of this surgery really clicked for me. This realization brought up so many questions. Why aren't we talking about the severity of this surgery? Why aren't moms walking out of the hospital with a prescription for physical therapy? Or at least a printout of recommended exercises? A sprained ankle is prescribed physical therapy. Why not a major abdominal surgery?

I'll cut these doctors a little slack though because their education isn't necessarily focused on post-baby rehab care. But, I'm hoping that changes supporting rehab care post-delivery happen sooner rather than later. And it's why we need to have more conversations about rehabilitation after pregnancy more often and f*cking loudly.

Pelvic floor (I'll talk more about this in chapter four) rehabilitation for moms after pregnancy and birth is equally as important as the prescription of physical therapy for patients after orthopedic surgery. In France, hospitals send moms home with what they refer to as a "cooch coach." Yup. These coaches are pelvic floor physical therapists, and they specialize in helping moms avoid symptoms like incontinence and pelvic organ prolapse. What a concept, right? Want to know what we offer in the US? The "husband stitch." That says it all right there.

The extent of care given to postpartum moms by the medical establishment in the US is limited and dismissive. I've heard from many of my clients that they were told to "just do your Kegels," or that surgery is the only way to fix their prolapse or incontinence issues. Some of my clients have received the same dismissive recommendations about their diastasis recti, a separation in the rectus abdominis muscles, the muscles you know as your "six pack." They are told that surgery is the only way to fix it. But I say bullsh*t. I know that these surgical interventions are not the only way because I've been able to help many women avoid surgery by rehabilitating their abdominal muscles. For moms, the movement practice of Pilates is especially amazing because it targets those all-important abdominal muscles that pregnancy and delivery can seriously compromise.

Let's look at the muscles that pregnancy and delivery impact.

These are the specific abdominal muscles that need rehabilitation, especially after a C-section surgery. Each of these abdominal muscle layers significantly stretches and weakens during pregnancy. And in the case of C-section surgery, they will have been cut through. Here are the muscle groups in order from the deepest to the most superficial layer of the abdominals.

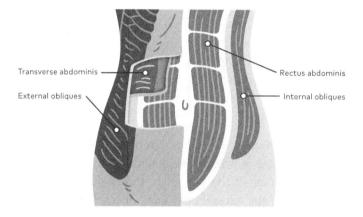

Transverse abdominis

External obliques

Rectus abdominis

Internal obliques

Transverse abdominis: This is the lowest and deepest of the abdominal muscles. Think of this one as your lumbar support belt. You've probably seen someone wear this type of belt while they were doing some heavy lifting at your local home renovation store. The transverse abdominis does exactly that type of work: it supports your lower spine and pelvis, minus the plumber's crack. The transverse abdominis is in the abdomen immediately inside of the internal oblique muscle. It is one of the innermost muscles of the abdomen, and it arises from the inguinal ligament, the iliac crest, the inner surfaces of the lower six ribs, and the thoracolumbar fascia. This muscle then inserts onto the linea alba, pubic symphysis, and xiphoid process (the bottom tip of the sternum).

Internal obliques: These muscles also support your spine. Without spine support, your back is required to do all the work. If these muscles are weak, your back will need to work extra hard, and that often leads to injury. The internal abdominal obliques are found on the lateral sides of the abdomen. They are broad and thin and form one of the layers of the lateral abdominal wall, along with the external obliques on the outer side and the transverse abdominis on the inner side.

External obliques: The large external oblique muscles cover the sides or waist of the abdominal area and sit on the top surface of the abdomen. Internal obliques are underneath the external obliques on each side of the waist. The external obliques originate at external ribs five through twelve and insert at the linea alba (the center of the rectus abs), pubic tubercle, anterior half of the iliac crest, and the front of the pelvic bone. These are your corset muscles. They hug your spine when you exhale, helping your back support your body. So, give your back a break and strengthen your damn abdominals.

Give your back a break. Strengthen your abs!

Rectus abdominis: Most people refer to these muscles as the six-pack abs. The rectus abdominis originates at the pubic symphysis or pubic crest and inserts at the xiphoid process and costal cartilages of ribs five to seven. It has a fascia layer, the linea alba, that connects the muscles and goes right down the middle. Sometimes the linea alba separates during pregnancy causing a diastasis recti.

Diaphragm: Pilates considers your diaphragm to be part of the abdominal muscles. In Pilates, breath plays a huge role in activating the abdominals and pelvic floor.

NOW THAT YOU KNOW what those ab muscles look like, let me tell you a little bit more about Pilates because it is the foundation of the Natalie Garay Methode.

Pilates: The Best Way to Rehabilitate

In case you aren't familiar with the history of this movement practice, let me tell you a bit more about its founder, Joseph Pilates. Born in Germany in 1883, Joseph Pilates was a sickly kid: he had asthma, rickets, and rheumatic fever. He used a lot of physical activity, such as gymnastics, diving, and skiing, to strengthen his weakened body. At one point, he was so strong and muscular that he worked as an anatomy model.

In 1912, Pilates moved to England. Because he was a German national, he was interned in a British camp at the start of WWI, which was when he started teaching other people his physical fitness techniques. During the last years of WWI, he helped rehabilitate wounded soldiers who could not walk. He added mattress springs to the patients' hospital beds to support and rehabilitate their muscles. This led to the creation of the Cadillac, or trapeze table, probably his most famous piece of equipment. In the early 1920s, he and his wife, Clara, moved to New York City and opened a studio (which is still there to this day) where they taught their body conditioning methods. Originally known as "Contrology," his techniques became known as the Pilates Method after his death in 1967.

Over the years, Pilates has become popular with dancers as a way of strengthening, stretching, and rehabilitating their dance injuries. And the method has only gained more popularity as celebrities began practicing it to achieve that long, lean dancer look. This form of body movement taught me about the importance of proper body alignment, breathwork, strengthening muscles, and the joy of moving my body. In any other type of exercise method or gym equipment, you're essentially targeting what I call the "bully" muscles. These are the big-ass muscle groups that people tend to overtrain to create massive, bulky muscles that leave them slow, inflexible, and incapable of optimal movement.

But Pilates makes it possible to reach and strengthen the deep muscles that no other exercise practice can do. Those tiny muscles that you find hidden under those bully muscles don't get enough credit for the work they do to keep us upright.

Pilates is the best way to begin rehabilitating your body. Pilates is for anyone and everyone, at any age and stage.

And I mean, *every*body. As a Pilates instructor, I can pinpoint exactly which muscles are weak and are causing the imbalance that leads to pelvic misalignment, back pain, neck pain, poor posture—you name it. That is the magic of Pilates—plus a good eye and twenty years of teaching experience. This is why I love Pilates. LOVE it.

In the next chapter, I'm going to share with you my experience of having a C-section. What I learned going through this experience is that this is no simple surgery— yet few of us receive aftercare instructions. Even if you had a vaginal birth, I still recommend you give this chapter a read because it contains some great information about rehabilitating your abs after pregnancy—and that applies to every one of us mamas. Let's get started!

YOUR EXERCISE GUIDE

Here are the Pilates exercises you will find in chapter fifteen that will help you strengthen your pelvic floor and abdominals.

- Pilates Breathing
- Pelvic Tilts
- Single-Leg Marching
- Pilates Tabletop
- Pilates Crawling

3

A C-SECTION IS A MAJOR F*CKING SURGERY

D O YOU KNOW WHY a C-section surgery came to be a procedure for delivering babies? Spoiler alert: a man invented it. Thousands of years ago, this procedure was used to preserve royal bloodlines. If a mother became ill and was in danger of dying, the baby was removed to save the patriarchal lineage.

Back then, a C-section was radical, but today, even though a C-section is still a major surgery, it's discussed like a straightforward wart removal and made out to be a simple, routine procedure. Why is that? I wasn't given the particulars or the step-by-step surgery details before having a C-section. Were you?

I was extremely curious about the whole experience involving my two months of bed rest and C-section, so I ordered my hospital reports. I have all 300-plus pages of detailed information about myself, my care, and the care of my tiny babies in the NICU. What I read and learned about my major surgery isn't for the faint of heart. Be warned: This may be a little graphic for you.

They start the procedure by numbing you from the waist down. I remember sitting on the operating table rounded forward while they stuck a needle into my spine. The anesthesiologist told me to let him know when I could feel any pressure. Every couple of seconds I would say,

"I can feel that." It was a weird, dull feeling of pressure into my spine.

I was given something for nausea as well, but that didn't work, because I threw that up shortly after lying down. Once I was down on the table, my arms were strapped down in a "T" position. The physicians placed a sheet between me and my lower half so that I couldn't see what was going on down below. Something that strikes me as odd now that I think about it.

When they began to cut through the skin, I could smell it because the doctor used something to burn through the skin. Let's just say that burnt flesh is not a scent that should be turned into a candle anytime soon. After they cut through the skin, they made a horizontal cut through the top layer of my abdominal wall and rolled back and clipped the muscles out of the way. They cut through more muscles, then cut through my uterus to retrieve my first little nugget. Two minutes later, they delivered twin B. I saw both babies briefly as the nurses held them hovered over my face, then took them away to care for them in the NICU. Once the babies were out, they stitched up my uterus and abdominals, then pulled my skin back together and stapled it.

Does that sound simple to you?

To the doctors who perform this procedure regularly, maybe it is, but that doesn't mean that this complex procedure doesn't take a toll on the body. And it certainly doesn't mean that physicians shouldn't advise us about proper rehabilitation and care afterward. The scariest part? I had a very touch-and-go moment after my C-section.

After my surgery, nurses took me to a room so that I could get some rest and recover from surgery. The nurses were coming in and out doing various things to care for me post-surgery while my parents sat bedside and watched me. At one point, while I was still talking with my parents, I started to fall asleep. I then stopped breathing, causing all my monitors and alarms to go off. Nurses and doctors rushed in to see what was going on. Hours later, after running every test and seeing every type of doctor in the hospital, they figured out that I was allergic to the morphine they had given me for the pain.

Here's some scary sh*t that you may or may not already know. Many women die at an alarming rate after a C-section (vaginal birth, too), especially women of color. In 2018 in the US, 17.4 out of 100,000 live births resulted in maternal mortality. However, according to the Centers for Disease Control and Prevention, Black women in the United States are more than twice as likely to die from pregnancy or childbirth-related causes than women of other racial groups.

Serena Williams made headlines after the birth of her child. After her C-section, she nearly bled to death. She explains that she didn't feel well and that something felt off. She told her doctors more times than she should've needed to before the doctors took her complaints seriously and listened to her concerns about feeling short of breath. Finally, the doctors discovered that she had a pulmonary embolism, which she describes as leading to a slew of health complications soon after. One complication was that her incision ruptured due to excessive coughing.

That surgery revealed issues with her blood clotting. All of these things could have killed her had she not spoken up and insisted that something felt off.

Since Williams is a champion athlete, I'm going to take a wild guess that she knows her body pretty damn well. She knew something was off, and yet she had to convince her doctors that she was right. Why wouldn't a doctor take Serena, of all people, seriously? Yet she had to tell her doctor multiple times that she needed help. She should have been taken at her word. Now, imagine if this wasn't Serena Williams. If we took away her fame, and she was a woman of color in the hospital trying to tell her doctor that something was off, I wonder how many times she would have had to speak up. This is why I believe it's important to know as much as you can about your body so that you can advocate for yourself when you need to.

Healing After a C-Section

Since you were likely not given a prescription for physical therapy after a C-section, you need to know the following things. Just after surgery, you'll want to keep an eye on your scar to make sure it's healing properly. If you notice any changes in feeling or color, get it checked out. You can also gently massage around the scar to help the healing process. You can do this soon after surgery and years later.

You can perform a gentle abdominal massage yourself or find a trained massage therapist who can help you. If it is not massaged, a C-section scar can become hardened and keloidal (when the scar overgrows tissue to protect itself). When a scar hardens, this causes the skin to fold over the scar to form a "shelf," which makes some moms self-conscious about their post-baby abs.

After surgery, scar tissue or adhesions may form over time and attach to organs or muscles inside your abdomen. Many of my clients have described a localized pulling sensation or a twinge when moving their body after a C-section, even years later. Adhesions are not necessarily bad if they aren't painful, but they are something to be aware of. Sometimes, these adhesions will adhere to organs and may even cause other issues. I'm pretty sure adhesions had something to do with a blocked bowel that sent me to the emergency room not long ago. My gastroenterologist confirmed this as a possibility after a recent routine colonoscopy. Here are a few ways to break up adhesions that may form after surgery.

MYOFASCIAL RELEASE

This type of massage releases adhesions formed after surgery. The technique focuses on releasing myofascial tissue, which can adhere to internal organs. This massage can also help create more energetic flow (something I'll talk more about in a later chapter) and your overall mobility. It can also help with the appearance of your scar. It may take a few sessions to fully break up the tissue, but it's well worth it to find a practitioner who specializes in working on scar tissue.

Physical therapy should be required after a C-section.

MOVING YOUR BODY

As simple as it sounds, just moving your body is a game-changer. If you are feeling up to it, go for a light walk as soon as you can after your C-section. But take it easy—no sudden or intense moves! In my opinion, Pilates is the best way to start moving your body. There is no other technique that will help your abdominals more than Pilates, especially when practiced on equipment such as the Reformer or Cadillac. Simple Pilates mat exercises can also be beneficial. At the end of this chapter, you'll find a list of exercises that I recommend to start your healing journey.

Rehabilitating Your Abdominal Muscles

Some time ago, a local ob-gyn reached out to me because he'd learned about the rehabilitative work that I was doing with my clients in my Pilates studio. When we met, he told me he was glad to know about my work and that he'd like to refer his patients to me. He agreed that rehabilitation after a C-section was important and he wanted his patients to strengthen their pelvic floor muscles first before suggesting they have surgery to fix their incontinence or prolapse issues (more about these things later). I can't tell you how relieved I was to hear this and to know that there are ob-gyns who are actively looking for ways to support their patients after they have given birth.

We chatted for some time, and I asked him questions about what he hears from his patients and how they're healing from their surgery. He shared with me that ob-gyn surgeons have changed their approach to C-sections. Now, instead of cutting through the abdominals to get to the uterus, they are separating the abdominal wall through the linea alba, the center fascia. This surprised me a little because even though I understood that surgeons were looking for a less invasive way to perform a C-section—and that is progress—honestly, I don't think having a diastasis recti after birth is any easier. That offers its own set of challenges, and I'll talk more about diastasis recti in chapter five.

In any situation, I am a firm believer that rehabilitation is still imperative. C-section surgery weakens your abdominal muscles, which can lead to a sh*t-ton of painful issues, such as back, hip, and knee pain, as well as poor posture.

Most people wouldn't necessarily connect the abdominals to being important for back, knee, or even pelvic support, but they are. It's one of the most important reasons I have for wanting to write this book. If all moms knew how much they need to restrengthen their abdominals after pregnancy, birth, and a C-section, it would change their lives!

In the next chapter, I'm going to talk about your pelvic floor and why it's just as important to rehabilitate as your abs after birth.

YOUR EXERCISE GUIDE

In chapter fifteen, you'll find specific Pilates exercises for rehabilitating your abs after a C-section. These are great ones to start with.

- Pilates Breathing
- Pelvic Tilts
- Single-Leg Marching
- Pilates Tabletop
- Pilates Crawling

4

WTF IS A PELVIC FLOOR, AND WHY IS IT SO IMPORTANT?

N 2015, I opened my first private Pilates studio in California. My sole purpose was to serve women who were experiencing physical issues related to pregnancy and birth. Up until this point, I'd spent the past ten years teaching in a few different studio settings. I never considered opening my own studio. It just looked like a sh*t-ton of work, from finding teachers and then subs for sick teachers to all the administrative work, and I didn't want any part of it.

But one day, while working with a client, we started talking about bladder leakage of all things. She continued to share a story about a horrific trampoline park experience she recently had while out with her kids. She'd driven her three kids and their friends a couple of hours south to enjoy a fun day out. After watching the kids enjoy themselves for a bit, she decided to join them on the trampoline and have some fun, too. But as soon as she took her first big jump, she emptied her bladder right there on the trampoline. Day. Over. She couldn't believe it.

We laughed a little about it, but then it hit me. Wait a minute. I've heard this story before and very similar stories of this kind many times over. Too many times. That was my light bulb moment. WTF is happening? Why is this happening, and why isn't anyone doing anything about it? Why are women experiencing this and living with it and laughing it off? Are we accepting this as the norm? It was a little confusing to me and made me mad, honestly. That's when I decided, not on my watch. I know how to fix this. Moms need to know that this *isn't* normal, and they do not need to live with it. That was the driving force for finally opening my own studio.

Today, when I see a mama with a couple of kids, the Pilates instructor in me starts thinking, "Two kids, huh? I wonder how her pregnancy was. Did she have a vaginal birth or a C-section? I wonder how she's feeling. Is she experiencing any pain? Bladder leakage? Oh my god, I hope she doesn't have a prolapse."

Would you run the other way if I stopped and asked you about your birth experience? I would love to ask each mama on the street these questions and direct her to the care that could help her. I'm a total weirdo, I know. So, instead of freaking moms out, I've put what I have learned in this book so you can read about it, use the tools, and pass it on to the moms in your life. Awkward interaction avoided.

Whether you've had one kid or ten kids, pregnancy and vaginal delivery stretch out your pelvic floor muscles. If you do not rehabilitate these muscles, you may experience bladder leakage or, worse, pelvic organ prolapse. How the effect of a weak pelvic floor shows up is different for all moms. Some will experience these symptoms soon after having kids; some experience it later in life but don't connect it to their pregnancy or birth.

Also, women experience multiple hormonal shifts throughout life, and these changes can affect the strength of their pelvic floor muscles. Pregnancy and birth represent just two of these changes. Other major hormonal changes happen during puberty, perimenopause (your thirties and forties), and then again when you finally enter menopause (usually in your early fifties). The muscles don't suddenly weaken when you hit menopause—this weakness is the sum of what's been happening over the years.

Your Pelvic Floor

So now you might be wondering, WTF is a pelvic floor? I am glad you asked.

The pelvic floor is a group of muscles that sits at the base of your pelvis and supports your pelvic organs—your bladder, uterus, and rectum. The bones of the pelvis that the muscles connect to are the ilium, ischium, and pubis. The muscles of the pelvic floor are stretched during pregnancy. Think of that commercial where water is poured onto a paper towel to show its strength. The towel stretches but doesn't break. Like that paper towel, the pelvic floor becomes more bowl-like and stretches with the weight of the baby as it grows. The pelvis also shifts and stretches as your hips widen in anticipation of delivery.

Want to know the boring names of these important muscles in the pelvic floor? The levator ani makes up part of the pelvic floor and supports the pelvic organs. The levator ani consists of three muscles: puborectalis, pubococcygeus, and iliococcygeus. The coccygeus muscles also make up the pelvic floor bowl that supports the pelvic organs.

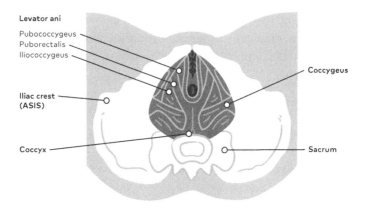

If you're a visual person like me, the image shown here of the pelvis will help you better understand what's going on down there. But just as a fun party trick, why not quiz your mom friends on the names of their lady parts? I would be surprised if someone shouted out "Pubococcygeus!" The good news is you don't have to have them memorized to know their importance, and you certainly don't have to f*cking live with a weak pelvic floor.

Now that you know how key your pelvic floor muscles are to helping you hold everything in, let me talk a bit more about the issues you might experience when your pelvic floor is weak. Be strong, mama, and remember—these are fixable.

Incontinence

Half of adult women experience urinary incontinence, and the prevalence of this problem increases with age. That's a lot of f*cking mamas who can't stay dry. Experiencing urinary incontinence while also parenting and running a business, a household, or all of the above is a lot to handle. So please don't. Incontinence tends to fall into two categories: stress- and urge-related incontinence.

STRESS-RELATED INCONTINENCE

I like to play a game anytime I'm around my sister, which is how many stupid things can I say or silly dances can I do to make my sister laugh until she pees? So far, the count is at three or four times. (That's what big sisters are for, right?)

Stress-related incontinence can happen when you sneeze, laugh, cough, or jump. Basically, all these activities put pressure on the pelvic floor muscles that keep the opening of the bladder closed, pushing urine out. The urine can't be held in due to weakened pelvic muscles. Are you familiar with the sneeze curtsy? This is a sudden crossing of the legs in hopes of keeping the tinkle from tinkling—something people with weakened pelvic muscles are all too familiar with. The exercises I've included in this book will help with stress-related incontinence. You can also look for a physical therapist who offers internal vaginal therapy and who can test your pelvic floor muscle strength so they can offer recommendations based on what they find.

URGE INCONTINENCE

My mom and grandmother had a habit of going to the bathroom before leaving the house "just in case." How many of you do this? The problem with this is you could be creating an unnecessary urge. Many women get the sensation that they need to pee suddenly more often than they would like. This occurs when you have a strong, sudden need to urinate that is difficult to delay. This can be caused by a few different things like an infection or a neurological disorder. Sometimes you may have the urge, and nothing comes out. Over the past several years, I've also learned that sometimes changes or injuries to certain brain regions can cause urge incontinence. This type of incontinence can also be a symptom of illnesses such as neurodegenerative disorders like dementia or substance-use-related injuries. If you suspect that your incontinence is more than stress-related, I recommend finding a qualified medical professional to help you find the cause.

MISALIGNED PELVIS

Sometimes, incontinence isn't entirely related to weakened pelvic floor muscles. A misaligned pelvis can also cause incontinence. Because the pelvis shifts and stretches so much during pregnancy and delivery, this can cause it to be out of alignment after the event. My first Pilates studio was attached to a chiropractor's office, and I loved it because we worked well together. He would see patients during their pregnancy and after. He would align them, and I would help them strengthen their hips, glutes, and pelvic floor muscles to help their pelvis stay in place. Seeing a chiropractor after birth to assess and realign your pelvis can be very helpful.

Pelvic Organ Prolapse

Remember the movie *Alien*? I do because I had to shut my eyes when the alien burst out of Kane's stomach—I couldn't handle it. Well, a prolapse of the pelvic organs is kind of like that except your pelvic organs are coming out of your vagina. Not a good look. And not fun to deal with daily.

Uterine, bladder, and rectal prolapse can occur when the pelvic floor muscles are weakened by vaginal delivery, pregnancy, and hormonal changes. Brace yourself because this next bit ain't pretty. Prolapses can happen at any age and any stage of your life. I've worked with moms who've experienced a bladder prolapse right after birth. I've also worked with a mom who experienced a prolapse of all three organs. Some moms won't experience or notice a prolapse until later in life. When this happens, it's often blamed on age. But, as I've said before, these things don't just show up suddenly; this condition has probably been a slow progression over time as a result of years without strengthening after birth.

UTERINE PROLAPSE

Uterine prolapse occurs when pelvic floor muscles and ligaments stretch and weaken and no longer provide enough support for the uterus. As a result, the uterus slips down into or protrudes out of the vagina. Uterine prolapse can occur in women of any age.

BLADDER PROLAPSE

This happens when the bladder drops down from its usual position in the pelvis and pushes on the wall of the vagina. In extreme cases, the bladder can drop right through the vaginal opening. It can be pushed back into place. In fact, I've had clients say that they've had to do this prior to their rehabilitative work. Just be aware that incontinence may precede a bladder prolapse.

URETHRAL PROLAPSE

This prolapse is less known and sometimes misdiagnosed. It results from the inner urethral lining protruding through the external urethral opening. Symptoms of a urethral prolapse can be urinary urgency and frequency.

RECTAL PROLAPSE

Rectal prolapse occurs when your rectum, part of your large intestine, slips down inside your anus. It's caused by a weakening of the muscles that hold it in place. Rectal prolapse may look or feel like hemorrhoids, but unlike hemorrhoids, it doesn't go away on its own. It can create a problem with controlling sh*t leaks. How's that for a description? I told you this wasn't going to be pretty. Don't fear! Let me remind you that this is fixable with pelvic floor muscle exercises.

Glutes, abs, and the pelvic floor: the power trio.

RECTOCELE PROLAPSE

A rectocele prolapse is when the rectum starts to make its way down the vaginal opening. The wall that supports the rectum and vaginal wall weakens, allowing the front wall of the rectum to sag and fall into the vaginal opening.

ALL OF THESE ISSUES aren't something to f*ck around with—this is serious stuff. If you don't do anything about your incontinence or pelvic organ prolapse, they will take a toll on your body and your emotional well-being. They may even affect your parenting or your relationships. You get the picture. So, what's a mama to do?

Think Beyond the Kegel

Wouldn't it be nice if you didn't have to plan your life around your bladder? Or get freaked out because your uterus could fall out of your vagina? Don't worry. I have helped thousands of mamas get back to their running routines, CrossFit workouts, and regular activities so that they do not have to double up on their black leggings, layer up with panty liners, or pack an extra pair of undies.

When it comes to incontinence, the Kegel practice seems to be the go-to suggestion by ob-gyns. In case you don't know what this is, a Kegel is an internal vaginal contraction. Kegel exercises for pelvic floor muscle strengthening were first introduced in 1948 by Arnold Kegel. Kegel designed the perineometer, also called the vaginal manometer (yep, *man*ometer, WTF?), to record the contraction strength of pelvic floor muscles and used it to guide participants to conduct the exercises correctly.

Many of my clients are told to practice their Kegels to fix the issues that a weak pelvic floor can cause or to consider a surgical fix. But surgery doesn't need to be your go-to solution. You can significantly improve or eliminate your incontinence and prevent pelvic organ prolapse with strengthening exercises. This isn't a quick fix though— it takes time, effort, and consistency—but it will work.

Although the Kegel is a convenient exercise that you can practice anywhere anytime, this single exercise alone isn't going to fix your problems. Why? Because all the muscles that I talked about in chapter two need to be involved in the strengthening process. I have designed the list of exercises at the end of this chapter, which you will also find detailed in part three, specifically to get that process kickstarted. As a side note, when working with new clients, I do have them initiate a Kegel contraction when trying to find and engage their lower abdominals (the transverse abdominis). But let that just be the start because you do need to think beyond the Kegel to rehabilitate your pelvic floor.

Put Your Ass Into It

Your butt is also a key player in supporting your pelvis. Your butt muscles are responsible for helping you stand and for supporting your knees, pelvis, and spine. Most people who have flat butts have back problems. Sorry, but it's true. But that's good news if you've been wanting to work on your butt. And no, getting a Brazilian Butt Lift will not help with this.

Here are the boring scientific names of your important butt muscles.

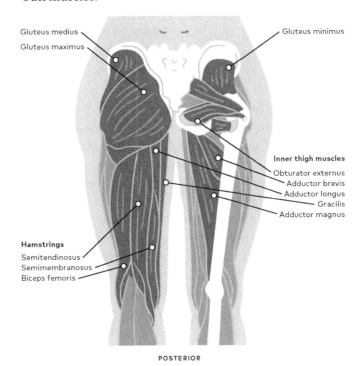

Gluteus medius

Gluteus maximus

Gluteus minimus

Inner thigh muscles
Obturator externus
Adductor brevis
Adductor longus
Gracilis
Adductor magnus

Hamstrings
Semitendinosus
Semimembranosus
Biceps femoris

POSTERIOR

Gluteus minimus: It's tiny, but holy sh*t is it mighty. No joke, if you never do anything else, strengthen this muscle and its big sister, the gluteus medius, because they are important hip stabilizers. Hip stabilizers hold your pelvis in place. While keeping limber is important, having an overly loosey-goosey pelvis has its drawbacks. Having an issue with one part of the body doesn't mean it stays within that part of the body. If your pelvis isn't stable, it can cause problems down to your knees and even to your ankles.

Gluteus medius: This sister muscle hovers over the gluteus minimus and gives it extra power. Again, the gluteus medius is a hip and pelvis stabilizing muscle.

Gluteus maximus: This big bad mama covers the other muscles. It is large and in charge and does a lot to support your back and pelvis. These plump muscles do the heavy lifting.

Hamstrings: Yup, hamstrings are also a player when it comes to your pelvic floor. Three muscles make up the hamstring: semitendinosus, semimembranosus, and biceps femoris. They connect to your pelvis and play a role in holding it together.

Inner thigh muscles: Your inner thigh muscles consist of five muscles, also known as adductors: gracilis, obturator externus, adductor brevis, adductor longus, and adductor magnus. They insert at the pelvis and make their way down your thigh bone. These muscles are important for pelvic stability and help facilitate pelvic floor contraction.

IT WON'T TAKE LONG for you to notice a difference if you make strengthening these muscles a regular practice. Again, this will be an ongoing practice. Once you learn how to fortify these muscles and gain some strength, that is only the beginning. To continue to reap the benefits of this newfound strength, you will need to move your muscles and continue to strengthen them regularly.

Avoid the Power Pee

Don't do it. If you pride yourself on being a fast pee-er, I'm sorry to tell you that this isn't a good thing. It means that you're pushing urine out, which means you're pushing your pelvic floor muscles down. This will stretch and weaken them. *¡No bueno!* When you sit on the can, relax, take a breath, and let the river flow. This also goes for going number two.

What About Yoni Eggs?

I get asked about these a lot (thanks, Gwyneth), so you'd think that just out of curiosity I would've tried them by now. But I have not, so I cannot speak from experience. I can only say, and I say this with caution, that they *might* be helpful in finding your Kegel contraction.

I've met several mamas who couldn't find their Kegel— they weren't sure if they were doing it "right." No judgment at all. It can be hard to reengage the muscles after having a vaginal delivery or even in general. When you shove a yoni egg up your vaginal canal, if you don't engage your muscles, the egg will fall out. So, if you aren't sure you're doing a Kegel contraction right, you may want to try a yoni egg. But there is also credible information out there that warns against using these, so just keep that in mind.

A better option to find your Kegel contraction is to pretend you're in an elevator and you have gas and need to hold it in. Begin the contraction from your anus and move the contraction forward. How's that for a visual?

IN THE NEXT CHAPTER, I want to take a closer look at your abs and specifically what happens when they separate during pregnancy. Whether this has happened to you or not, the information about your abdominals will be helpful.

YOUR EXERCISE GUIDE

I've seen Pilates exercises work wonders for my clients, so in my opinion, this is the best route to take when rehabilitating your pelvic floor. And remember, always think beyond the Kegel. I've helped thousands of women improve their symptoms and their quality of life by teaching the following simple and effective exercises to strengthen their pelvic floor. What do you have to lose (except maybe an organ or two)? You can find these exercises in chapter fifteen.

- Pilates Breathing
- Pelvic Tilts
- Bridging
- Single-Leg Marching
- The Clam Series
- Pilates Tabletop
- Pilates Crawling

5

WTF IS
A DIASTASIS
RECTI?

RENEE CAME to me at the referral of a midwife at her ob-gyn's office. She had two kids, and, at the time, her second child was about a year old. Her main complaint? "I still look three months pregnant!" Renee's two pregnancies and an abdominal wall separation had weakened her abdominal muscles and caused her linea alba to separate, which gave her the appearance of having rounded abdominals—a pooch, if you will.

Maybe you've looked at your profile in the mirror after pregnancy and thought, "Holy hell, I still have a bump?" Or maybe you've discovered a soft spot where you can press your fingers through your abs and thought, "WTF is this fresh hell I have to deal with?" Well, that's diastasis recti (DR).

So, what exactly is DR? Well, there's a line down the middle of your top abdominal layer called the linea alba. (I know these terms aren't all that exciting, but bear with me because I spent a lot of time and money memorizing these boring names.) The linea alba is a fibrous structure that runs down the midline of the abdomen. Fibrous means filmy; it's like that weird white layer you can find on a raw chicken breast. When your abs are stretched to the max during pregnancy, the linea alba can separate, and it separates even more after multiple pregnancies.

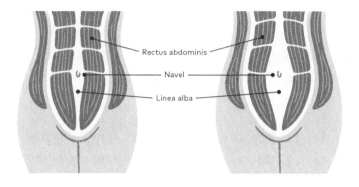

DR bothers most moms for the appearance it causes. But more importantly, it can trigger a chain of painful events when you don't take care of it. I'm not here to shout out, "We want pre-baby body!" Instead, I want to help you feel your best, gain strength, and eliminate pain so you can function at an optimal level. (Good news, though, you'll also like the bonus effects.) To do that, you need to know the details of how this abdominal separation happens.

WTF Happens When You Don't Fix Your DR?

During pregnancy, the abdominal muscles can separate down the center because, hello, have you ever seen something grow this big so quickly? Your abdominals are stretched to the max, and some of us nearly pop. Like, for real.

There are ways to test if you have DR, but you may already know something is not right in your abdomen. If you have DR, you may have noticed something trying to escape your body through your abdomen when you get out of a chair or your bed. I joke, but this isn't something to ignore. If you're not affected by the appearance, that's great. But where DR is concerned, you *should* care about what it can mean for the rest of your body. Everything in your body is connected, and one weak link can ruin your day.

Let me break it down for you.

If your abdominal muscles have separated, whether that's right in the center, just below the belly button, or right under your rib cage, this means that your muscles are not working at full capacity. And that means that your other muscles are working overtime. More importantly, it means your back is pulling double, and maybe even triple, duty.

Remember in school when you'd get put into groups to complete a project? There was always one person who did all the work, and everyone else pretended to look busy. Well, that's your spine. Let's call her Sheila. Sheila is pissed. She's doing all the work. She needs help, and she's not afraid to tell you.

Sheila's going to b*tch and moan and let you know how she really feels. And she's going to do this by giving you some low back pain or some sciatic pain. Yup, that's Sheila saying, "HELP ME!" She may also throw in some neck ache, chronic hip pain, and a pinch of knee pain. Sheila's tired of holding up your entire body; it's a hell of a lot of work, and it's time to lend her a hand. Help a sister out by strengthening your abdominals and eliminating that separation.

Your abdominals wrap around Sheila the spine and give her a nice big bear hug, supporting her while helping

Surgery is not the only way to fix a diastasis recti.

her hold up the rest of your body. Your head alone weighs about eight pounds; that's a lot for your little vertebrae to support.

Ever notice your posture? It's your abdominals that keep you upright. Weakened abs cause the shoulders to round, which makes the head lurch forward. Weakened abdominals lead to a whole chain of nasty events.

Your hips? Yup, they're a part of this, too. If you have hip pain, it's likely due to a misaligned pelvis. That misaligned pelvis will then press on a nerve, sometimes sending pain down your leg. A misaligned pelvis can also cause knee issues. Everything is connected, and one missing Jenga-like piece can cause the whole structure to collapse.

Strong Abs Relieve Back and Neck Pain

Pregnancy and birth take a monumental toll on your body. When your abdominal function is weakened from a DR, even holding a baby can be a challenge. That simple movement will require more work from your back and eventually lead to achy hips, neck pain, and too much weight and pressure on your spine.

Weak abs contribute to poor posture, and poor posture puts more pressure on the spine, causing compression to your spinal discs and your internal organs. Compressed internal organs make it more challenging to breathe fully, which can lead to poor oxygen flow and result in less clarity of mind. Poor posture also results in your heavy head lurching forward, which puts strain on your upper trapezius muscles in your shoulders and causes chronic neck pain. See how it's all connected?

Let's get back to Sheila, remember your friend, the spine? One of the main jobs of your abdominals is to hug and support your spine. Strong abdominals relieve back pain and prevent disc-related issues, support the pelvis, alleviate knee issues, correct poor posture, and improve the quality of your life overall. So, I'll repeat it for the crowd in the back: strengthening your abdominals is *muy, muy importante.*

Zip Up That Abdominal Gap

When it comes down to it, you have three options for fixing your DR:

- You can either live with it (I don't recommend this).

- Repair it surgically (I don't recommend this either, at least, as your first resort).

- Or you can rehabilitate your muscles with Pilates (ding, ding, ding, I highly recommend doing this!).

Some of my clients have said that when they asked their doctor about their DR, their doctor dismissed it as just a result of pregnancy and recommended surgery as their *only* option to repair it. But surgery *isn't* the only way to fix an abdominal separation. There is another way! (Picture me yelling into a megaphone.) This fix takes time, effort, and consistency, along with a few simple exercises that I'll share with you at the end of the chapter.

Ob-gyns don't always recommend rehabilitation as a first stop for body issues related to pregnancy. Some are simply not familiar with the kind of rehabilitation available. But I've noticed that ob-gyns who work closely with doulas or midwives are more informed about other methods for care and rehabilitation. So, if you did have a doula or midwife assist you during pregnancy, it's worth asking for their recommendations. If not, you can still reach out to one for support.

LET'S GET BACK TO my client Renee. After working with me for several months, she was able to eliminate her abdominal separation and build back her core strength through regular Pilates sessions. Eventually, she was able to hold her kids with more ease and less pain. And she was definitely pleased to be pooch-free.

But correcting abdominal separation isn't a one-and-done thing. Renee worked hard. She came to my studio at least once a week for more than three months, several times with her babies in tow. (I was more than happy to see them and hold them if needed. I'm quite the multitasker.) She also practiced her exercises regularly at home. You need to move and exercise your muscles regularly, especially when you're trying to build strength. If she wasn't doing her homework, she wouldn't have seen results as quickly.

You should expect to put in solid, consistent work for three to six months to experience a significant change in your body strength. That's not to say that you won't see or feel a difference sooner; Pilates is amazing in that way. One of Joseph Pilates's famous quotes is, "In 10 sessions you will feel the difference, in 20 you will see the difference, and in 30 you'll have a whole new body." Joseph Pilates was a f*cking genius in my opinion. And his method is life-changing.

I'll repeat this over and over: Pilates is the best method for any rehabilitation. I've helped clients rehabilitate hip, shoulder, knee, and back surgeries with Pilates. But it's especially great for getting back into a movement practice and restrengthening the abdominals after pregnancy, delivery, C-section, and a diastasis recti. It's gentle, effective, and tailored to what you need specifically. Your rehabilitation time will depend on the severity of your separation, but, if you stick with it, you'll be amazed with the outcome. Just keep the end goal in mind—you are strengthening your muscles so you can get your life back.

AT THE END of the day, I want you to have optimal energy, brain power, and bandwidth to accomplish all your daily tasks and big life goals. This will require more energy, and that all starts with the foundation, your body strength. Funny thing, the more you move your body and build strength, the more energy you'll have.

YOUR EXERCISE GUIDE

I have included exercises in chapter fifteen that *will* help you fix your DR slowly but surely. For this specific issue, I recommend these exercises:

- Pilates Breathing
- Pelvic Tilts
- Single-Leg Marching
- Pilates Tabletop
- Pilates Crawling

However, in the beginning, you'll want to avoid exercises that make it challenging to maintain abdominal engagement. The last thing you want is for the gap in your abs to expand, so make sure that whatever you're doing, your gap is as closed as possible. Exercises that could be counterproductive in this instance are crunches or anything with a sit-up motion. Plank is another exercise you'll want to avoid in the beginning since you're likely unable to properly engage your abdominals at that stage.

PART TWO

MORE THAN BONES AND MUSCLE

6

WTF IS AN
ENERGETIC
BODY?

W E'RE NOT just a compilation of skin, bones, and muscles. There's more to you than just your physical body and more to us that we can't even see. Now is the time to get curious about what is making us not feel like ourselves. Sometimes we just can't pinpoint what it is that's bothering us. That's when we have to dig a little deeper and learn about the other parts that make up who we are—the unseen things that we don't often talk about, but should be.

Let's start with the energetic body. There's an invisible energy that runs through us that affects our daily actions, our mental and emotional well-being, and our overall health. Who knew, right? Here's the weird part: illness often shows up on an energetic level before it does in the physical body. And for mamas, it's especially important to show your energetic body some love along with your physical body. I first learned about the energetic body when I started practicing yoga. But let me rewind and tell you what really went down at that time, the whole ugly story about when and how I was feeling my worst.

In 2011, I was living in Los Angeles as a solo mama doing my best to keep my sh*t together while raising my three adorable little nuggets—the twins were nine at the time, and their sister was seven. I was in major survival mode trying to keep them fed, get them to school, and make it to work on time. Talk about struggling. I was doing it with a capital S. I felt like sh*t. I was unhappy, unmotivated, and feeling just plain blah. I wasn't having any fun. I didn't know what to do with myself. I wasn't sure how to pull myself out of this funk. But for my girls' sake, and my own, I knew I needed to get it together.

Since I was teaching Pilates, that was the only thing I knew to do. I mean, it *was* what I was preaching to my clients every damn day. Move your body—you'll feel better. Move your body—it will give you more energy. Move your body—it increases endorphins, endorphins make you happy, and "happy people just don't shoot their husbands." (My favorite quote from the great Elle Woods in the movie *Legally Blonde*.)

So I took my own advice and started to move my body. I wanted to do something I enjoyed so that I would stay motivated, which was Pilates. But I knew I needed to find someone to keep me accountable and to keep me consistent because I couldn't rely on myself to stay focused. I mean, clearly, I wasn't making the time in my schedule; I was more focused on getting to work, doing the work, and then getting back to the girls. All necessary life tasks, of course, but not entirely exciting or energizing. So, I signed up for a yearlong membership at a Pilates studio close to home. This was a huge time and financial commitment for me, but I was more than ready for it. Deciding to commit to something is the first step, and the rest is follow-through. But you must decide to commit first.

One of the perks of signing on for a yearlong commitment meant that I got first dibs on the classes. This allowed me to sign up three times a week at 9:00 a.m., one of the more popular class times. The timing of this class fit perfectly with the morning school drop-off schedule, which meant that I had zero excuse to not take my happy ass straight to Pilates.

I did it. I went three times a week for eleven months. Now that's commitment. You should have seen my bod! But that was *nothing* compared to how energized and joyful I felt. I was practically walking on a f*cking cloud. I felt a new sense of motivation, and it sparked so many creative ideas. This girl was on fire. I was looking and feeling *caliente*!

I was *so* on fire that I was ready for a change of pace and scenery. I decided to move out of LA and head north to the central coast. The move left me just a month shy of completing that twelve-month membership. (Don't worry, they made sure I paid for it.)

This move was an incredible change for me and for my girls. They loved their new little school on the bluffs overlooking the water—who wouldn't? They could even ride their bikes to school. And I was soaking up my new slow-paced, beach-bum life and feeling really good. With this newly found energy and sparkling confidence, I decided to start my own business, a virtual Pilates studio that allowed me to teach inside my beachside abode. Yup, I was teaching virtual Pilates in 2012 long before the pandemic hit and the world transitioned to living on Zoom.

That one tiny decision and commitment I made to myself for my mental and physical well-being put a lot of new and amazing things in motion for me. But most of all, it got me out of my dumpy funk and reignited some passion for life in me.

My real healing journey had begun. I had no idea how tense I had been up to that point, or how much sh*t I had been holding on to. It's amazing what getting out of your daily chaos can do for clarity. The girls and I would take walks on the beach each day after school; it was so calming and grounding. The change from living in a big city to a small-town beach community was such a nice shift. The pace was slower, the people seemed kinder, and everyone was just... happy.

But I started to miss my movement practice that I had started at that Pilates studio in LA. So, I found the cutest yoga studio just walking distance from our beach house and signed up for a membership. At this point, I wanted to keep this fire lit. I'd never practiced yoga before. I didn't know much about it except that people who loved it, really loved it, and they loved to tell you all about it. I just wanted to keep moving.

I did pretty well throughout my first class. I followed along, attempted the poses, and enjoyed learning something new. It felt great, which is always a bonus, and the instructor was kind and gave me a few pointers here and there. Toward the end of the class, I was feeling good as I stretched and activated new muscles. Then, after all the hard work, the instructor had us lie down and relax in Savasana (corpse) pose.

Suddenly, out of f*cking nowhere, tears. Tears came streaming down my cheeks and pooled in my ears. I lay

Your inner world reflects your outer world.

there thinking, "WTF? What is happening? Why am I crying? There's crying in yoga?"

I cried for the duration of Savasana. I released something that clearly needed to go. I had no idea what it was, but it just came out. I knew from my Pilates and dance background that movement was powerful and that it could cause an emotional release, but I was not expecting this. Something in me broke wide open, and it was coming out all over my mat in my first yoga class.

When class ended, I rolled up my mat and made my way up to the front of the class and hugged the instructor and thanked her. I was a little dazed and definitely confused. But also, lighter. I walked home slowly while wondering what had just happened.

I went back every day during the first week of my new membership and each class ended the same way, with tears streaming down my cheeks and pooling in my ears. It was f*cking incredible. This is when I realized that there's a lot more going on in the body than many of us realize. I continued to practice yoga for a few years and learned a lot about the body's energy systems—and eventually what all that crying was about.

Your Energetic Highway

In her book *Anatomy of the Spirit,* Caroline Myss explains that there are five layers to the body: physical, energetic or etheric, emotional, mental, and spiritual. All of these layers are interconnected and react to each other through meridians or chakras, which are called subtle energy bodies. The medical field has called this energy system the biofield. Any block in the energy flow can show up in a few different ways, from physical pain to emotional symptoms like lack of motivation or depression.

I like to visualize the energetic body as a highway that runs through the body. Picture cars on the highway moving in a loop from the feet, up the leg, to the top of the head, and back down and around in a racetrack formation. When there's an accident, it really f*cks up the flow, which causes stagnation in the body.

Ancient Indian and Chinese cultures understood the idea of the energetic body long ago. You may already be familiar with the energetic body if you've taken a yoga class, and the teacher told you to pull up your *mula bandha*. And you, like me, were probably thinking, "WTF is a moolah-banda?" This is a yogic practice of drawing the root chakra up and in. The root chakra is energy that lives at the base of your pelvis. This energy is often associated with feeling a sense of safety and security and feeling grounded.

Although yoga has been around for thousands of years, it has gained a huge following and popularity in the wellness and holistic community. Some people have mistaken yoga for a religion, but yoga breath work and movement were originally practiced more for clarity of mind, flexibility, and improved well-being. Yoga helps strengthen and protect the spine, while the breath work in yoga plays an important role in the energetic body. Moving through various poses with a focus on your breath can bring you into a meditative state.

As the popularity of yoga has exploded, the chakras are probably now the most well-known energetic body system. Most people who know about the chakras are familiar with the seven listed here along with their Sanskrit names and associated colors:

- Root chakra: *Muladhara* (red)
- Sacral chakra: *Svadhishthana* (orange)
- Solar plexus chakra: *Manipura* (yellow)
- Heart chakra: *Anahata* (green)
- Throat chakra: *Vishuddha* (blue)
- Third-eye chakra: *Ajna* (indigo)
- Crown chakra: *Sahasrara* (violet or white)

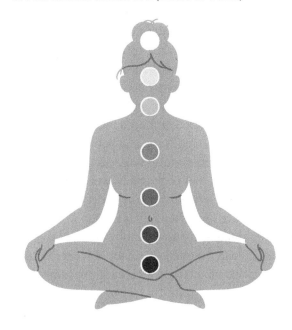

Simply put, the chakras work as energy distribution centers. When your life force energy is balanced, it can flow easily through channels in your body—known as the *nadis* in yogic practice or meridians in Chinese medicine—and into the chakras for distribution. When your circulation system is open and in flow, it creates a life force energy in you that helps you maintain overall happiness and well-being.

When energy is stuck in a chakra, you may feel fatigue, brain fog, or a lack of motivation. These are just some of the minor symptoms of blockage that you shouldn't ignore because the symptoms tell us that if we don't get moving and take better care of ourselves, something more serious could show up, like chronic illness and disease. Yes, this unseen sh*t is serious stuff.

OVER THE NEXT few chapters, I'm going to explore the first three chakras in your energetic body—the root, sacral, and solar plexus chakras—because pregnancy and delivery directly affect these three. Then I'll talk about the remaining chakras and how they play a role in your daily well-being. As you read through each chakra description, take mental or physical notes about the symptoms that may reflect your current or past situation. Check out the tools in chapter sixteen to help you assess your energetic body.

GROUND AND CALM THE F*CK DOWN:

THE ROOT CHAKRA

CAN'T TELL YOU how many times I've heard my post-pregnancy clients say, "I just don't feel like myself anymore." It makes sense. How could you? You go through an unbelievable transition during pregnancy and delivery. Everything has changed and shifted, right down to each cell in your body. The childbirth experience is an extreme transformation in who you are.

Dr. Oscar Serrallach, a functional medicine doctor, wrote about "watching his wife wither away" after each pregnancy in his book, *The Postnatal Depletion Cure*. He'd seen this from a distance in his patients, but when he watched it happen in his wife over the span of a few years, he began to do more research about how the pregnancy process takes such a huge toll on a woman's body. He says that it's possible that up to 50 percent of moms may face postnatal depletion to some degree.

Years ago, I interviewed practitioners, physical therapists, and other healers, as well as moms who shared their birth experiences and life after pregnancy and birth on my podcast. One mother shared her experience of psychosis after having her baby, and that interview has stuck with me over the years. This mom was so altered by giving birth that she spent time in a facility to rehabilitate and recover. At the time, I thought, "Holy sh*t!" I simply couldn't imagine that a woman could experience this extreme of a reaction from having a child. But over time, as I've learned more about the post-baby body and what the body goes through to create a healthy baby and more about the brain (after my mother passed away from dementia and my daughter experienced a substance-induced psychosis), this scenario makes so much more sense to me.

The body goes through such a massive change and transformation during birth and pregnancy that it can literally send you into an extremely different and altered state. We saw this sequence of events play out publicly with Britney Spears. Knowing what I know now, I believe that part of her psychotic episode was due to the massive changes she experienced when she had her kids so closely together. Of course, I'm sure there's most likely more to it than that, but that experience alone might have been enough.

That is part of the reason I talk so much about the root chakra with my clients; it is located directly at the base of your pelvis, at the perineum, right by the baby-maker. This is where all the action happens before pregnancy, during pregnancy, during the birthing process, and after. Since the root chakra is located at the base of the pelvis, it is directly affected during pregnancy as the pelvis shifts and then again during a vaginal delivery.

Your root chakra energy can be affected if you experienced tearing during delivery or after an episiotomy and now have a scar. Imbalances that could show up include feeling ungrounded, insecure, and anxious. You may even experience an imbalance as a lack of resources, both materially and emotionally. Physical symptoms can include chronic back pain, autoimmune issues, incontinence, and chronic urinary tract infections (UTIs).

The Qualities of the Root Chakra

The color red represents the root chakra, and the qualities of the chakra are:

- Safety
- Security
- Passion
- Abundance

When You Need a Recharge

You may have noticed in your transformation to motherhood that you've lost a sense of passion or that you don't feel as stable or secure. Maybe things are just a little wobbly. You're just not yourself, that's for sure. You may not realize what the culprit for the feeling is. All you know is that something feels off in you and in your zest for life. If you have this vague off-kilter sensation, it's most likely because your root chakra could use some shaking up. Having a sense of knowing and security is pretty damn important, especially for you mamas if you want to feel more grounded so you can take on the fabulous f*cking goodness of motherhood each and every day.

Root,
ground, and
calm the
f*ck down.

Your root energy is attached to your lower extremities and organs so when energy is blocked or unbalanced in the root chakra, this can show up as physical symptoms such as:

- Lower body issues in the lower back, legs, feet, knees, and the base of the spine
- Constipation and bowel issues
- Weight gain or loss
- Weakened immunity
- Fatigue and/or insomnia

WTF, right? These are not simple aches and pains that you can ignore. So, what do you do? My go-to practices of Pilates and yoga are the best practices for reigniting energy flow. Both modalities place a huge focus on breath, physical form, and being mindful about your movement. Not to mention that both practices engage the pelvic floor muscles and strengthen your hips. Another cool (or not so cool, depending on how you look at it) thing that I learned in yoga was that we store our negative emotions in our hips. Hence my crybaby experiences that first week of yoga.

To get your root energy moving again, take a look at the assessment questions and the exercise for the root chakra that I've recommended in chapter sixteen.

NEXT, WE'LL LOOK AT how your creativity and sense of worthiness are connected to your pelvis and sacral energy.

IGNITE YOUR BOWL OF CREATIVITY, SELF-WORTH, AND MOTIVATION: THE SACRAL CHAKRA

HAVE HAD three major life shifts that were the result of a committed and consistent movement practice. The first time was in 2008, when my client at the time, actor Kaley Cuoco (how about *that* name-drop) invited me to her spin class in Hollywood. The first class was hard as hell, and I nearly threw up, but I was immediately addicted and scheduled my life around my new spin class addiction. I loved going so much; I couldn't stop talking about it. I cannot tell you how much those classes changed my life. They changed my attitude, changed my body, and changed my work and home life dramatically. I left each class feeling so incredibly pumped, energized, and excited about life every single time.

The second major life shift came after committing to the Pilates practice three times a week that I shared earlier. I was stronger, more energized, and creative ideas were a-flowing. I had a renewed feeling of motivation. Life had new meaning, and I was excited about it. It inspired my decision to move out of LA, gave me ideas for a new business, and I was no longer such a moody mama. Oh, and let me just add this mini bonus—I looked GOOD! Not that that was the goal, but it was a welcome byproduct.

And the third shift in my life, of course, was as a result of my yoga practice that I told you about in chapter six. Here's why all those three stories created so much shift in my life.

The sacral chakra is associated with creativity, self-worth, motivation, and overall enjoyment of life. This energy is located inside your pelvic bowl, the exact place where our reproductive organs are located and where we happen to house and create humans, sometimes two (or more) at a time! That's a whole lot of responsibility for one little ball of energy. That is why I talk about the sacral chakra so much with my clients.

Did your creativity vanish after you had your kids? I've heard from so many clients that they've lost their sense of motivation and their creativity, and they don't even care for sex anymore. *¡Ay, caramba!* We need to get these things back in order, sister. It's not okay to let everything just slip away. No f*cking way. Maybe you didn't even realize your creativity had drained away. That disruption of these unseen forces is the invisible reason why we just don't feel right after pregnancy and birth. You can't quite put your finger on it, but you know something is off. And because you can't really see it or name it, that's often the reason why some medical professionals dismiss your bad feelings as "normal."

Pregnancy and delivery tend to throw everything out of whack inside you. Some women bounce back faster than others, but all women who go through these massive body changes need to look at the reasons why they might not feel like themselves anymore. Those feelings play a huge role in how we exist daily. Read that again: this energetic

Power to
the pelvis,
your bowl
of creativity.

block has everything to do with how you act, think, breathe, and BE in the world.

Why wouldn't you want to pay attention to and adjust that?

What about the physical manifestation of stagnant sacral energy? Get a load of this sh*t: Prolapse, incontinence, spinal pain (between the lumbar and sacral spine), low libido, and even autoimmune disorders are symptoms of unbalanced sacral energy. And that's just the start. That's a lot of serious stuff related to this invisible energy running through your body.

By activating or reigniting energetic flow in your sacral chakra, you will feel more energized and improve your creative expression and your overall enjoyment of life. And if you're not here to simply exist, I believe this is an absolute must.

The Qualities of the Sacral Chakra

The color orange represents the sacral chakra, and the qualities of the chakra are:

- Creativity
- Inspiration
- Motivation
- Self-worth
- Relationships

Read through this list and take a mental note if you feel like any of these things have taken a hit since you had kids.

If you feel less motivated and less inspired, or that your sense of self-worth has plummeted, don't worry; these things can all be improved to their regular function, or even better.

When You Need a Recharge

When the energy in your sacral chakra is depleted, it may show up physically in the following ways:

- Prolapse
- Incontinence
- Spinal pain (between lumbar and sacral)
- Low libido
- Autoimmune disease

Again, you should not take any of the above lightly. Working on your physical symptoms will require both physical strengthening and energetic shifts. In part three, you will find exercises for both. In chapter fifteen, I recommend these in particular:

- Pilates Breathing
- Pelvic Tilts
- Bridging

The Grounding Meditation in chapter sixteen will help you reboot your root and sacral chakras.

IN THE NEXT CHAPTER, we're going to talk about reigniting your power and finding your inner badass.

STAND IN YOUR F*CKING POWER, SISTER:
THE SOLAR PLEXUS CHAKRA

'VE WATCHED the entire *Grey's Anatomy* television series more times than I should probably mention. It's sort of a self-soother for me. There are a few things I love about this show. A woman created it, there are several women on the show's writing team, and many of the directors and producers are women. At one time, a client of mine was a writer on the show, and she happened to be an emergency room doctor. In front of the camera, the show highlights badass female doctors in leadership roles as chiefs of each medical department.

I love seeing women taking their place in the world, even if it is just a TV show. We need to see this. We need to see women represented in high-achieving roles, especially women of color. I love that my daughters have seen this and that they can see themselves represented in these shows. My daughter Nia came home from high school one day to tell me that her biology teacher was impressed that she answered a tough question correctly. After asking my daughter how she knew the answer, the teacher laughed when Nia replied, "*Grey's Anatomy.*"

In one of my favorite episodes, Dr. Amelia Shepherd, chief of neurosurgery, is about to take down the worst brain tumor she's ever seen. She's studied it, practiced on a brain model, and dreamed about the tumor for weeks. She's prepared herself, and she *knows* she's the best surgeon for the job. When the day of surgery arrives, after scrubbing in and just before entering the operating room, she takes her power pose. Fists on her hips, chest out, chin up, standing tall, she is standing in her power.

That's what I picture when I talk about the third chakra, also known as the power chakra. It's located at the solar plexus, just above the belly button, and it's the source of your power, will, and confidence. This is the center of your creation! But the act of creating a human shapes and shifts the flow of power in that chakra. No wonder you may not feel like yourself after pregnancy. You may find that your confidence is now low or has even gone into hiding altogether.

If you're not feeling strong, confident, and on fire, it's time for a recharge. You need this energy to keep spinning because it's what keeps you feeling empowered to go after your goals and desires.

And that's where yoga and Pilates come in. Both movement practices connect you to your core, your power center. You can't help but walk out of a Pilates session feeling like a f*cking badass. It makes you stand taller, feel stronger, and if your belly could, it would be shooting out the most glorious golden light and yelling, "Out of my way, people. I'm coming through!"

The Qualities of the Solar Plexus Chakra

The color yellow represents the solar plexus chakra, and the qualities of the chakra are:

- Self-esteem
- Will
- Power of transformation
- Gut instinct

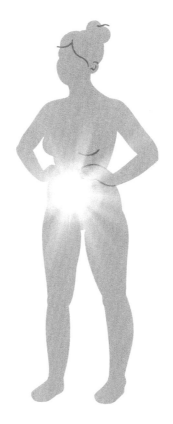

Strike a pose
and remember
who the
f*ck you are.

Ask yourself if you've noticed any shifts in your self-esteem, your sense of will, or your desire to do things. When the solar plexus is dampened, it's like we simply exist without a sense of direction or purpose. I don't know about you, but that sounds like a wasted life and just plain boring. Ask yourself if you've lost your sense of self and purpose. Have you lost or forgotten about any dreams or goals? What would it feel like to go after them again?

When You Need a Recharge

When your solar plexus energy isn't flowing, it can show up as the physical symptoms listed below. Many of these conditions are serious, and you should obviously not ignore them.

- Chest pain
- Stomach pain
- Anxiety
- Intestinal contraction
- Painful sensations in the upper abdomen
- Severe abdominal pain

But on top of seeking medical help for these issues, and moving your body, you can also start to reactivate the energy of your solar plexus chakra through the breathing practice I've suggested in chapter sixteen.

IN THE NEXT CHAPTER, we'll move to reviewing the upper chakras: the heart, throat, third eye, and crown.

TAP INTO YOUR HEART, VOICE, INTUITION, AND GUIDANCE:

THE UPPER CHAKRAS

ABOVE THE root, sacral, and solar plexus are four more chakras that are just as important and indirectly affected by birth and pregnancy. Think about the energy channels like a hose with a kink in it. When energy is not flowing through the lower chakras, that energy is also blocked from flowing through to the upper chakras, resulting in a big ol' traffic jam in your chakra highway.

A disconnect between the lower half and the upper half of the body can make someone appear flighty or "out there" because they aren't grounded. When you're grounded, you're able to move through life with clarity, guidance, and a strong sense of knowing who you are and what the f*ck you want. Every one of us is naturally intuitive, but it's harder to tune in to that intuition when you are not grounded. Once the energy is flowing in your lower chakras, then you can connect to the goodness of the upper chakras.

Access Your Compassion and Empathy: The Heart Chakra

The color green represents the heart chakra, and the qualities of the chakra are:

- Love
- Compassion
- Joy
- Empathy

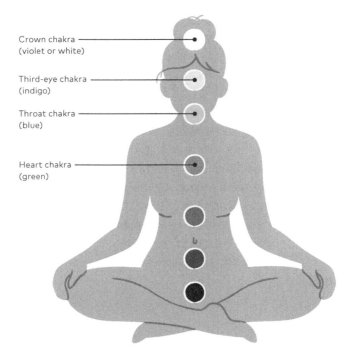

Crown chakra
(violet or white)

Third-eye chakra
(indigo)

Throat chakra
(blue)

Heart chakra
(green)

This energy system lives smack dab in the middle of the chest, obviously. It's the center of love for ourselves and for others and where you feel compassion, empathy, and forgiveness. I've said this about every energy system, but this one is *muy importante*. If we could consistently live in love, empathy, and compassion, how much would half the stuff we worry about daily really matter?

Know anyone who could use a little more heart chakra energy? Kidding. Not kidding.

I have this interesting (weird?) thing that I do when I hear about another tragic event on the news of somebody hurting another person for reasons I will never understand or of a crime someone has committed. I think about this person as a baby or toddler, like an actual tiny being. That's not who they were when they were born, is it? I wonder, what was this person's life like? What were the circumstances that formed this person? How is this person feeling inside? Are they hurting? Are they just hungry? Need love? What led this person to be this person who's now on the news for making a terrible decision? I'm not ignoring the event, but I have compassion for the person behind the act.

This may be extreme, and I'm not asking you to do the same, but if we led with love, curiosity, and compassion daily, would the world be a better place for it? I think so. I choose love, dammit.

Speak Your Needs, Wants, and Dreams: The Throat Chakra

The color blue represents the throat chakra, and the qualities of the chakra are:

- Self-expression
- Expressing creativity
- Communication

The energy of this chakra gives us the power to express inspiration and to use effective communication. I feel like moms and women in general don't use their voices enough. Many of us stifle asking for what we want and what we need. As moms especially, we should be able to ask for what we need. Let's stop suffering in silence and speak up. Stop trying to do everything yourself, and ask for help. Do you have big dreams and goals? Share them. Speaking things out loud gets the ball rolling, and it lets people and the universe know exactly what you want. Use your voice, and don't hold back.

Tap Into Your Inner Knowing: The Third-Eye Chakra

The color indigo represents the third-eye chakra, and the qualities of the chakra are:

- Intuition
- Clarity

You are
naturally
intuitive.
Just tap in.

- Imagination
- Spiritual connection

This chakra is related to perception and awareness. Think of this energy as the ability to think from a different perspective—this is your inner knowing. Although physical and emotional awareness are amazing tools, your inner knowing makes things work out so much more easily and calmly, and it allows you to move through life with clarity because your authentic truth guides you from the inside. When you take the time to sit and listen, your intuition and inner knowing will answer your questions and offer guidance.

Access Your Divine Guidance: The Crown Chakra

The color violet or white represents the crown chakra, and the qualities of the chakra are:

- Gratitude
- Acceptance
- Divine guidance

This chakra taps into your spirituality and awakens your enlightenment. The crown chakra is your direct connection to divine guidance. Whether in prayer or meditation, visualize the crown of your head opening and allowing guidance to come down from above. Continue this visual and take that energy down your spine and through your limbs to your feet and into the earth, allowing you to feel guided and grounded.

In chapter sixteen, I've shared a link to a full-length guided grounding meditation that you might find helpful for activating all your chakras.

AFTER READING all of this information about energy and the chakras, you might be thinking, WTF? Don't worry, I did, too, at first. If a system like the energetic body plays such an enormous role in our health, lifestyle, and overall quality of life, why isn't this more mainstream or more widely discussed? I haven't the foggiest, as my grandmother would say, but that's why I wanted to share what I've learned, plus a few tools to get you started on your own knowledge journey.

None of the tools that I am sharing with you in this book will be a one-stop shop. But each tool will help support the healing of your entire system. I want you to have this information so that you can be fully informed about what's happening in your body and have a base of knowledge to choose from to help yourself if you decide to. Isn't that better than asking WTF and being left in the dark or feeling hopeless, like there's nothing you can do?

IN THE NEXT CHAPTER, I'm going to discuss another unseen system that I think you should know about because, just like the energetic body, it can have a big impact on your well-being.

EVERYTHING IS CONNECTED: THE BRIDGE OF WELL-BEING

EVERAL YEARS AGO, I attended a conference designed for budding and successful entrepreneurs in Portland, Oregon. The speaker lineup was incredible. Each speaker filled me with excitement and inspiration. At the end of each day, I left the theater with pages of notes full of ideas, motivation, and even new friendships with other crazy thought leaders who no longer wanted to live the rat race.

One memorable speaker discussed her time as a very successful CEO running a large corporation. But her crazy work life made her sick, literally sick, and eventually she was diagnosed with a serious illness. The constant daily stress of her job had shown up in her body, and she had a choice to make. She could either stay in this stressful job and continue to get worse and die or leave and find a new life. She chose to quit her job, start her own business, reduce her possessions, move into a tiny home, and completely simplify her life. The decision to completely change her life saved her life. This story has stuck with me for a long time. I was inspired by the speaker's complete life transformation and the fact that she was able to renew her health.

Many years later I began to learn more about the multiple connections between our inner and outer worlds. It's mind-blowing how so much of what we do and what we breathe in every day affects our health and well-being. Our environment, our work, the people around us, the food we eat, and even the things we watch and listen to, all play a role in our emotional body and health.

Nobody wants to be ill. Nothing seems to be worse than being laid up on the couch or in bed with a terrible virus, or something worse. Our whole world seems to stop when we're sick. And for moms? Holy sh*t. If mom's out of commission, nothing gets accomplished. At least in our house, it didn't.

Nothing else seems to matter when you become ill, especially if you receive a serious diagnosis. Things come to a complete and screeching halt, and everything turns inside out because at that moment what was once important no longer f*cking matters.

Here's what I propose. Let's not wait for this kind of huge wake-up call before deciding to take care of your emotional well-being. What does that look like? Let's get into it.

Your Cells Have a Memory

On her website, Professor Laura Bond explains: "You are an emotional body. You were born with a body primed and ready to express your needs through emotions, and they influence all you feel, think, do, and say. Everything you encounter triggers your emotions, and then influences your health, relationships, perspective and perception of the world."

I love Bond's description of the emotional body as intimately connected to the mental and the physical body. It's important to know about how our thoughts, emotions, and experiences can affect our health. Your thoughts deposit a sh*t-ton of weight on your well-being and your health. Your thoughts and emotions can make you sick, literally. There's a connection between what you think and what you are feeling and your physical symptoms. You've probably heard some form of the saying, "What you think, you become." Well, here is how that works.

Your body is made up of cells, and each cell has a memory that holds all of your emotions and experiences—the good, the bad, and the ugly. When you experience something unpleasant and painful and you don't take steps to heal yourself, the stored imprint can compromise your emotional well-being or factor into illness and disease. Your body keeps the score of your experiences throughout your life, and these experiences build on each other over time. If you stack up negative experiences and never release them, they can become heavy and drag on you mentally and physically.

Back in 2020, I had the opportunity to participate in a program presented by Suzy Batiz, creator of Poo-Pourri. Her program had nothing to do with business in the way we would think it should, but the information she shared, according to her, was the foundation of building a successful business. One of my favorite sentiments of hers is that what resides in your inner world can create your outer world. In other words, whatever sh*t show is going on inside you is going to show up as a sh*t show in your

Your body keeps the score.

life. Or the reverse: whatever good stuff is vibrating inside will show up outside. The bottom line is that you need to be mindful of what's going on inside of you and with your thoughts.

Yes, I know. It's so easy to get wrapped up with life, but being busy and stressed nonstop sends your body into a state of chaos. Your chaotic mind sends a stress signal to your body, which increases your stress hormones, which then causes inflammation in your body and lowers your vibration. Inflammation in your body is like a slow ember waiting to be stoked by more stress into a full-on sh*t show of a fire in your body. Your low vibrations are a breeding ground for a sh*tty life or sickness.

For me, this looks like a skin reaction. I get eczema spots on the backs of my legs when my body is inflamed. When it's really bad, like right now while I'm writing this book, it itches like a b*tch. When this happens, I start to ask myself questions: How can I destress? What can I eliminate from my diet that's inflammatory? What additional tools can I try that will help me? What's stressing me out, and what can I do about it? Usually, my go-to tools include seeing a chiropractor and an acupuncturist. Both practices always help with reducing my stress and calming my body the f*ck down.

But you can also think of the mind as a tool in the process of calming yourself. Your mind, or an initial thought, kick-starts the process and sends the signal to the body. We've all experienced a day when something goes sideways, and it sends you into a sh*tty mood. This bad mood makes everything seem like it's f*cked. Or is it? It all depends on how you choose to move forward. You can certainly stay in a sh*tty mood and chalk it up to "just your luck." But that's only asking for more trouble. That's a magnet drawing more sh*t to you. Sh*tty just got sh*ttier. That's the power of the mind. You just created that. But imagine if you focused on the good stuff in your life instead. Check out chapter seventeen for an exercise that will help you access your current vibrational state and help you raise those vibes if you need to.

We're Always Vibing

Did you know that we all vibrate at various frequencies? Yes, your mood actually has a number attached to it. Our emotions can generate a frequency, and the lower, or less desirable, the emotion, the lower the frequency.

In my most recent classes on my journey to becoming a naturopathic doctor, I took a general physics and chemistry class. This sh*t was like learning another foreign language, especially for this dancer/Pilates instructor/creative mama. But I loved it and thankfully not-so-gracefully ended the classes with Bs. In both classes, we talked about frequency. This isn't some fluffy bullsh*t; this is science. The level at which we vibrate all begins with a thought; that thought creates a vibration, whether low, medium, or high; and the people around you can feel that vibration.

In the cone shown below, you can see the vibrational frequency number in hertz, which I think is the coolest thing ever. Joy, sadness, and shame—they all have a frequency level associated with them. If you've ever heard someone say raise your vibration, they may not have known it, but it is actually a frequency that you can change. And one way to raise those vibes is to be grateful.

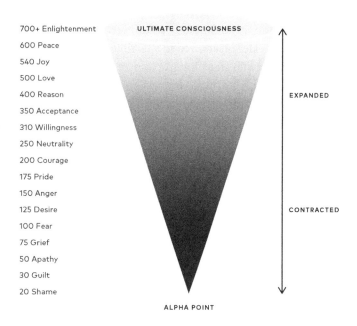

OMEGA

700+ Enlightenment
600 Peace
540 Joy
500 Love
400 Reason
350 Acceptance
310 Willingness
250 Neutrality
200 Courage
175 Pride
150 Anger
125 Desire
100 Fear
75 Grief
50 Apathy
30 Guilt
20 Shame

ULTIMATE CONSCIOUSNESS

EXPANDED

CONTRACTED

ALPHA POINT

Gratitude Counts

Have you heard about the life-changing effects of a gratitude practice? This practice may sound simple, and even silly, but gratitude is a high-frequency emotion that creates joy and expansion in our body and cells. We do operate like magnets, whether we're attracting things to us or repelling things from us; that attraction all depends on your vibrational frequency.

Take, for example, author and researcher Dr. Joe Dispenza. Dr. Dispenza, a trained chiropractor, has shared his incredible healing story on many podcasts, and it never gets old for me. It's a fantastic example of how powerful our minds are. He was injured in a terrible accident during the biking part of a triathlon. As he was making a turn at an intersection on his bike, a four-wheel-drive Ford Bronco going fifty-five miles per hour hit him from behind. He landed hard on his back and broke six of the vertebrae in his spine.

His surgeons wanted to fuse his spine by placing a rod through it. But rather than having the surgery, he decided to use his mind to heal himself. Sounds crazy, right? He spent hours a day visualizing a perfectly healthy and healed spine. Can you imagine? He describes how he would sit for hours and simply visualize each part of his spine and body in perfect form. And incredibly, in just three months, he says that he was on his feet, back to work, and exercising again! I'm still stunned but inspired every time I hear him tell the story. It's an extraordinary example of determination and how powerful the mind is.

But I would get so distracted, you say. You're not alone in that. Dr. Dispenza talks about how he'd have to start over with his visualizations if he got distracted or if he let a negative thought slip in. Calming the mind might come easier for some than others—it takes practice.

Take a few pauses throughout the day to stop and assess your state and thoughts. Can you shift them toward a more positive thought? It seems so simple, I know, but it does immediately shift your state and your vibration. Here are some examples to try.

If you're feeling worried, try shifting your thoughts to: "There's nothing to gain from worrying. Everything is working out the way it should."

If you're feeling angry, shift your thoughts to gratitude for what's right in front of you.

If you're feeling hopeless or exhausted, maybe you just need to take a nap, drink some water, and remind yourself that tomorrow is a new f*cking day.

This list of thought shifts gives you an idea of how to figure out what sh*t needs to be shifted or released and how to do it.

IN THE NEXT CHAPTER, we'll talk about why it's so important to release your sh*t. Before we do that, in chapter seventeen, you'll find a quick exercise to help you assess what you might need to let go of. The Emotional Vibration Assessment exercise will help you pinpoint any lingering low-energy feelings or thoughts that you need to address. Time to let that sh*t go, sister.

RELEASE
THAT SH*T

WHATEVER WE'RE holding on to will eventually rear its ugly head. Whether that's through an angry outburst, crying like a baby in yoga, or becoming physically ill. So instead of waiting until an unfortunate event, take a look at some ways to release any sh*t that's stored in your body unnecessarily.

There are many great tools for helping you release stored emotional sh*t, raising your vibration, and feeling lighter. I have tried all of these energetic modalities and use them as my go-to list of healing tools. They are worth trying to see if they will work for you:

- **Acupuncture:** for ensuring a smooth flow of energy throughout all meridians and for reconnecting the "upper and lower" bodies

- **Chiropractic care:** for realigning your pelvis and calming your nervous system

- **Reiki:** for energy balancing and grounding

- **Somatic therapy:** for releasing and creating energy flow

- **Myofascial release:** for breaking up scar tissue and creating energy flow

- **Massage:** for energetic flow, detoxing, and relaxation

- **Infrared sauna:** for detoxing, mental clarity, and energetic flow

You don't have to do all of these practices, but find what works for you, experiment, and create a list of modalities for when you're not feeling great, like an emergency support list.

These supportive modalities are good to have when you're smack in the middle of a sh*t storm because that is precisely when you may lose common sense and not know what to do. Your "In Case of Emergency" list will come in handy when that happens. One modality that works for me and that I have incorporated into my rehabilitation method is flower essence therapy.

Flower Essence Therapy

A few years ago, I was on a retreat in Montecito, California, with some mystical and magical mamas. We stayed in a gorgeous house for four days, taking in the greenery and sun while setting intentions for our upcoming projects and life.

My room was in the coziest little guest house just off the main house—perfect for this little introverted crab. I like quiet, and I like my sleep. I'm usually the first one to retire, even when I'm on a retreat. But it so happened that I had a wonderful roommate who was the sweetest, gentlest woman from LA. Janice was a flower essence therapist who spent time supporting mamas as a doula. She created magical tinctures to heal them on an energetic and cellular level.

When she learned about my Pilates practice and how my focus and expertise was helping women rehabilitate their physical symptoms after having kids, she started to tell me more about these magical potions that she created. I had never heard of flower essences before. I was, of course, familiar with essential oils, but these are completely different. Today, many people are familiar with Bach flower essence remedies and its most popular tincture, Rescue Remedy. This remedy is also a flower essence, a combination of flowers for when sh✳t hits the fan.

Flower essences are unscented homeopathic remedies that offer gentle healing. They help you feel more grounded and can help your body release all those emotions that you store in it over time at the cellular level. I was completely intrigued and loved the idea that these flower tinctures helped women feel safer and more supported. So intrigued that not too long after meeting Janice, I took her flower essence therapist certification program and her subsequent master training program so that I could have this new skill and tool to offer my clients.

I began making healing tinctures for my clients, which, when combined with their movement practices, would accelerate their healing. Their Pilates practice was already working to strengthen their muscles and move energy through their body, but the addition of the tinctures helped them feel more grounded while gently supporting the release of anything they were holding on to unnecessarily after pregnancy and birth.

Using Flower Essences

Flower essence remedies are taken sublingually, usually in a concoction of natural spring water and a smidge of brandy to preserve the remedy. Apple cider vinegar can also serve as the preservative instead of alcohol. Flower essences are created using the vibration of the flower and fused into water under the sunlight. Each flower offers its own unique healing power. I currently have a collection of about ninety flower essences, all very supportive of specific needs in their own magical way.

Flower essences perform their magic on an energetic and cellular level, using the vibrational energy of the flower for healing. I think people often dismiss how powerful and healing plant medicine is. Plant medicine is all that people had for many years to use for various ailments.

I've listed some of my go-to flower essences below. I use these flower essence remedies often with my clients as well as in my Theramist products, which are therapeutic mists made with essential oils and flower essences. (You can check them out at youneedtherhappy.com. I think they're pretty awesome.)

These essences help calm down your system while also bringing you back into your body. They offer protection, grounding, and peace.

NATALIE'S FAVORITE FLOWER ESSENCES

Lemon balm	Helps you with deep relaxation
Borage	Strengthens courage and lightens a heavy heart
Lovage	Creates a deeper connection to the divine feminine
Angelica	Offers protection during times of stress and change
St. John's wort	Offers energetic protection and mood enhancement
Lady's mantle	Supports clarity of purpose and a sense of self
Yarrow	Offers energetic protection
Missouri primrose	Helps with recognizing worthiness and a sense of power

Move Mindfully: Go Slow to Go Fast

A few years ago, some friends created a documentary called *Slow Is Fast*. I remember thinking, "huh?" As I wrote this book, this title popped into my head because it reflects a core theme of this book: moving mindfully is more effective and productive than living at warp speed in chaos to get sh*t done.

When I get busy or stressed, I tend to take more shallow breaths or hold my breath altogether without realizing it. When I became aware I was doing this, I found an app that led me through a five-minute breathing practice to help me take longer and deeper breaths. The practice of taking long, deep breaths calms my nervous system, sends oxygen to my brain, and helps me think and see more clearly. This practice isn't just beneficial to me; it's something everyone can benefit from.

When you take the time to stop, breathe, and rest, you're better equipped to function properly and keep your sanity. Let's be honest, when mama's not happy, ain't nobody happy. You're not doing anybody any favors when you continue to run on overdrive and run yourself ragged.

What if you focused on your health and well-being first? What if you took time in the morning to journal a bit, meditate, or even do a short breathing practice before jumping out of bed? These simple practices can create more peace and relaxation in your mind and your body and send out positive emotional ripples for the rest of your day. I truly believe that this can set a tone for a happier and healthier mama—and a happier and healthier home.

When you take the time to meditate or journal, you learn how to filter out the least important tasks and take care of the more important things in your day. This act of prioritization creates a magical effect that eliminates the less important things, making your day that much lighter.

Taking care of yourself, even in some small and mindful way, will help you accomplish so much more than if you hustle your way through life. The stories I've shared with

Let that sh*t go!

you here show that the emotional body really is something to take care of. I'm not saying that you need to spend five hours a day to take care of yourself, just a few minutes. You are worth it, and it will change everything for the better.

Listen up, sister. I know I've just thrown a lot of information your way. You may be thinking, "Well sh*t, where do I even start?" But don't you worry. We're going to take this healing journey in small doses. And I'm going to walk you through it step by step.

This is stuff I've learned and practiced for more than twenty years. It will take time to develop a routine and find a tool kit that works for you. Just know that solutions will shift and change every few years, too. So don't stress about it. You don't need to go vulva-to-the-wall and practice everything all at once. Some of these tools may not even pertain to you. But I want you to have all the information in case you ever need it or in case you have a friend in need.

In part three, I've put together a step-by-step guide to help you get started. You'll find all of my favorite tools and exercises to help you feel stronger and more energized in no time. You can forget about the endless YouTube and Google searches. I've done that for you and tested all these remedies on myself and my clients. And I'm not finished learning yet. You can keep up with me on Instagram at @nataliesayswtf as I make my way through school to become a naturopathic doctor (class of '29!). I'll be sharing what I learn along the way about hormone health, brain health, and my current obsessions relating to women's health.

Mamas, this is your time. You must put your health and well-being first.

Start slow.
Listen to your body.
Don't ignore your symptoms.
Get curious.
Ask questions!

And for the *love of everything*, please talk to your friends and other women about what you're experiencing. Don't suffer in silence. There will always be someone who's experiencing what you're experiencing, too. Women need to talk about their incontinence issues and not just joke about it; we need to share what's worked for us and what hasn't. Share the resources and don't let anyone say, "It's just part of being a mom" ever again.

Reclaim your health. Reclaim your vitality. Don't fall for the bullsh*t that your health doesn't matter after having kids or that your symptoms are a trophy of being a great mom. You can and should come back to your full strength and power. You're needed at your best. This world needs you. Your community needs you. And goddess knows your family needs you.

I have goals. Lots and lots of f*cking goals, pages of them. I can't possibly accomplish them if I'm limping through life lethargic and sick. Neither can you. So, I'm training for life, sister! This is how I want you to think about it, too. Who knows how long we'll be here, but while we're here, let's make sure we're operating at full capacity.

What you do daily and how you take care of yourself will not only help you thrive, it will also encourage and teach future generations. Taking care of yourself doesn't just benefit you, it helps your family and your community. The kids are watching you and taking note; there will be a ripple effect. When you're happy, people will see it, feel it, and be inspired by it.

Here's to feeling your f*cking best!

A TOOL KIT
TO REBOOT
YOUR BODY

13

POWER-UP YOUR HEALING JOURNEY: A STEP-BY-STEP QUICK-START GUIDE

I'VE DESIGNED my rehabilitation method to look at the whole person and body. Throughout the book, you've been given the opportunity to look more deeply into WTF is really going on with your body and with your life. I think it deserves repeating: what's going on in your inner world is expressed in your outer world.

Making a thorough assessment and following that up with a practice of subtle changes can lead to massive shifts in your life. This approach has affected my life as well as the lives of my clients. Over the next several weeks, I'd like you to follow the list below and use these steps as your guide. Build on them as you go. My clients tell me they can hear my voice throughout the day, so as creepy as it may seem, think of me repeating these steps to you as your remote guide.

Step 1: WTF Is My Body Trying to Tell Me?

At the beginning of this book, I talked about how awareness of what your body is saying is the first plan of attack. Keep this in your mind as a starting point and journal about it. Write down what you think your body is trying to tell you with any aches or feelings: WTF is my body telling me? If your journal isn't handy when you want to write your answers down, take a note on your phone.

Take a few minutes a day to do the Initial Body Check-In in chapter fourteen, as well as the Daily Quick Scan exercise in the same chapter.

Step 2: WTF Can I Do to Feel Better?

Once you've figured out what your body is trying to tell you, make a list of go-tos that will help you feel better. You can choose from a list of my favorite modalities that I listed in chapter twelve as a starting point and see which practices serve you best.

_____

_____

_____

_____

_____

_____

_____

Next, run through the Body and Mind Scan exercise found in chapter fourteen.

Step 3: Where the F*ck Is My Road Map?

It's time to implement your practices slowly. Start by choosing the Pilates exercises from chapter fifteen that support what your physical body needs from a rehabilitative perspective. Write the exercises down below and practice them regularly while also implementing the other modalities that you decided will help you out, such as acupuncture or chiropractic care (see the list in chapter twelve). List those practices below as well. Tips for success with fitting in appointments: Make sure they're convenient, prepay, schedule them ahead of time, and add them to your calendar. These are the guaranteed ways to help you make it happen.

_____

_____

_____

_____

_____

_____

_____

_____

_____

_____

Start slow;
get curious;
ask questions.

Step 4: When the F*ck Should I Check In?

Take a moment to check in and see if your body is responding to the movement or therapies you've implemented. This could be after a week or a month, but it's important to take note of any changes and improvements along the way. Notice whether you're less fatigued, less irritable, or if you're sleeping better. These may seem like minor shifts, but, over time, these subtle shifts will add up to enormous improvements. List how you're feeling and what improvements you're feeling.

After one week

_____

_____

_____

After two weeks

_____

_____

_____

After a month

_____

_____

_____

Step 5: WTF Do I Really Want?

Part of feeling better means you may feel more excited about doing new things or accomplishing goals. You can do this more effectively when your body is cooperating and functioning optimally. If your body is starting to feel better, and you're feeling more energized, you can now start to shift your focus to future endeavors.

Go back to the goals that you listed from chapter one in the Training for Life section. You can number these goals in order of importance if that's helpful and list them here.

1   What is it that you want to do in a day?

_____

_____

2   What do you want to accomplish in a month?

_____

_____

3   How about in five to ten years?

_____

_____

4   What will you need to be able to complete it?

_____

_____

Step 6: WTF Am I Waiting For?

Now get after it, sister. Pick a goal from your list, write out the steps that you need to take to accomplish it, and start taking small steps to get there. Complete it, celebrate (a very important step), then pick another one, and repeat the same steps.

Over time, these steps will come to you more easily and naturally. It all starts with feeling your best so that you can have the energy to live life. Like I said, I'm training for life. I want to feel my best, and I want to increase and maintain my energy and strength so that I can function optimally each day. I may not hit the mark every single day. It's important to remember we're not trying to push through anything—rest is important, too. But we have to become aware of what's going on inside first.

14

RAISING BODY AWARENESS EXERCISES

'D LIKE TO OFFER some exercises that will help you start listening to your body—because that is where it all starts.

Your Initial Body Check-In

You can kick-start body awareness by asking some of these simple questions when you're feeling off. Use these questions as journal prompts, or just sit quietly and close your eyes after each question while you wait for an answer.

What are you feeling? (List your current emotions.)

1 _____

2 _____

3 _____

4 _____

5 _____

What aches? (List all the "things" that are talking to you.)

1 _____

2 _____

3 _____

4 _____

5 _____

What is your current energy level? (Rate from 1 to 10.)
If your energy level is low, list the reasons why your energy is at this level.

1 _____

2 _____

3 _____

4 _____

5 _____

What would help improve your energy level? (If needed.)

1 _____

2 _____

3 _____

4 _____

5 _____

How do you want to feel on a regular basis?

1 _____

2 _____

3 _____

4 _____

5 _____

What can you shift in your daily habits/routine
that would help you feel the way you want to feel,
if anything?

1 _____

2 _____

3 _____

4 _____

5 _____

Body and Mind Scan

You can do this two-part practice alongside the previous
one, and it might help you with filling out your answers. I
like to do this practice in the morning before starting my
day. It's simple and only takes a couple of minutes. You
can do it in bed before you get out of it or while sitting in
a comfy chair.

PART 1: YOUR BODY

Sit comfortably. Inhale deeply and then exhale. Next, close your eyes, sit tall, and take your attention to the top of your head. We're going to do a full-body scan, starting from the top.

Slowly, with your eyes closed, check in with your body and make your way down. Start by relaxing your face, then shoulders, and then check in with all your body parts as you continue to make your way down to your feet.

What parts of your body are talking to you? Any aches or soreness? If so, what can you do to ease them? Maybe some light stretching or a hot bath?

Now check in with your energy level. How are you feeling? Sluggish or vibrant? If you're feeling sluggish, what can you do to support yourself to feel more vibrant? It could be eating something clean and green or inhaling a vibrant citrus scent.

Check in with what's going on around you. Is your space quiet or chaotic? If it feels chaotic, think about what tiny shifts you can make to create more ease and peace.

PART 2: YOUR MIND

After you've checked in with your body, check in with what you are thinking. Your thoughts can affect your mood and zap your energy without you even realizing it. If you want to have the best day possible, you want to dump bad sh*t as soon as you can.

Here's a way to help that process: Is there anything negative swirling around in your head? Write it down in a journal. Just start writing, and dump it all out.

Reclaim your health and vitality.

Once you've written it down, ask yourself what this thought is and why it's in your head. Where did it come from? Is it true?

Then continue with the "why" questions until you get an answer or until you feel less dominated by the swirling thoughts dragging you down.

Daily Quick Scan

Once you've done your initial scan and made your assessments, you can also do a quick version of this scan each day. Take five minutes to do a body scan and visualize each part of your body strong and pain-free. Think about how thankful you are for your body and its ability to move you through life.

PILATES-BASED EXERCISES

THE FOLLOWING Pilates-based exercises will help you gently activate and strengthen your deep core and glute muscles to help you rebuild your physical foundation. I've chosen these exercises to help you start slowly by activating the deeper muscles. From there, you can build on that foundation. These are simple yet effective exercises that I walk all my new and established clients through. They are gentle enough for beginners but just as effective for moms who have already started a movement practice.

Give them a try. Just remember that should you ever feel any pain or discomfort in your back or otherwise, adjust as needed or stop. You never want to "work through" the pain. If you need more guidance or have questions about whether an exercise is right for you, email me at wtf@nataliesayswtf.com, and I'll offer more specific instruction.

Pilates Breathing: A Pelvic Floor and Abdominal Strengthener

Anyone can do this exercise! The Pilates breath is one of the most important parts of the entire Pilates practice. Essentially your breath is like gas in your tank. The breath engages your abdominal muscles so that you can perform the exercises effectively and accurately without injuring yourself. Simply exhaling engages your abdominal muscles, and, believe it or not, doing this multiple times strengthens those muscles.

You can practice this exercise either sitting upright in a chair or lying on your back with your knees bent.

Start by wrapping your hands around your waist, with your thumbs at the back, fingers in the front.

Take a gentle inhale, then slowly exhale with a slight "shhh" sound coming out of your mouth as if you're quietly telling someone to shush. This is a gentle breath, so make sure you're not overtightening your jaw or mouth.

Notice if you felt your waistline shrink as you exhaled. I like to describe this as pretending like you're wearing a corset, and it is being tightened as you exhale.

Try it again. And then practice this simple inhale-exhale exercise ten to fifteen times all the while feeling your abs engage and relax. Continued practice will strengthen your abdominals.

That's it! So easy, so gentle. And you don't have to do a million crunches to gain strength.

Pelvic Tilts: A Pelvic Floor and Abdominal Strengthener

This is another simple but effective Pilates exercise that will help you reactivate and strengthen your abdominal muscles after surgery.

Start by lying on your back on a mat, bend your knees, and keep your feet on the floor. Place your hands around your waist again so that you can feel your muscles engage when you exhale.

Place a small (nine-inch-diameter) ball between your knees to help with pelvic floor muscle activation.

Your pelvis should be in a neutral position. What that means is that you should not feel the small of your back flat to the floor, and it should not be overly arched.

Exhale gently as you use your lower abdominal muscles to tilt your pelvis toward you so that the small of your back flattens on the floor.

In this exercise, make sure that your abdominals are doing the work and not your legs or back. This is a small and gentle movement that you should feel in your low, deep abdominals between your hip points. You may not feel this right away, so keep repeating the motion to "wake up" your abs.

Bridging: A Hip Stabilizer and Glute Strengthener

This exercise is another great, gentle way to activate and strengthen your abdominals. Again, it's super simple but very effective. You may feel the effects of each exercise differently, so for this reason and for the purposes of variation, practice this and pelvic tilts as part of your exercise routine.

Start in the same position as you did in the previous exercise, lying on your back, knees bent, feet on the floor, and hands around your waist or on your hip points.

You *can* come back to your full strength.

Place a small Pilates ball (nine-inch diameter) between your knees to help with pelvic floor muscle activation.

Inhale gently and then start your pelvic tilt again. This time, as you exhale and tilt your pelvis toward you, lift your glutes slightly off the floor. Don't come up too high and keep your ribs closed. Once you are in the bridge position, keep your abs scooped as if you were making a bowl out of your abdominals.

Inhale at the top of the movement, and then exhale to engage your abdominals to roll back down, one vertebra at a time.

Do this five to ten times, again focusing on using your abdominals to initiate and complete the movement.

Single-Leg Marching: An Abdominal and Glute Strengthener

Start with breath work: Sitting or lying down, place your hands around your waist and exhale to feel your waistline shrink. Repeat ten to fifteen times to feel your abdominals contracting.

Next, move to a single leg lift (marching): On your back, bend your knees, and place your feet hip distance apart. Place your hands around your waist, exhale to feel your abdominals engage, and then use your lower abdominals to lift one leg slowly.

Place the leg down. Repeat the same movement on the other side. Repeat five to ten times on each side.

The Clam Series: A Hip Stabilizer and Glute Strengthener

This exercise looks exactly like what it's called. Imagine your legs are the shells of a giant clam opening and closing.

Lay on one side with your elbow under your head. Stack your legs with your knees bent and in line with your hips.

Keep your feet together as you lift the top knee as you exhale. You should feel your outer hip (gluteus minimus) get tired after ten reps.

Repeat on the other side.

CLAM WITH LEG CIRCLES

Lay on your side. Stack your legs with your knees bent and in line with your hips.

Keep your feet stacked together and lift the top leg/knee in line with your hip as you exhale.

Hold it up and pretend you have a pencil pointing forward from your kneecap. Make small circles with your knee. If your circles are too big, you won't be able to keep your pelvis steady.

Repeat ten times in each direction.

Pilates Tabletop: A Pelvic Floor and Abdominal Strengthener

You do this Pilates tabletop exercise on your back. Do not confuse it with the yoga version of the tabletop move, where you're on your hands and knees. This simple exercise will let you know right away how weak your abdominals are.

If you have DR, you'll want to make sure that you're able to keep your separation closed in this position. If holding both legs in tabletop is too challenging, try holding just one leg up for a few seconds. Alternate legs and build up to being able to hold both legs up.

Lay down on your back in a supine position. Bend each knee to place each foot flat on the floor, feet slightly separated. Place your hands around your waist so you can feel your abdominals engage with the exhale.

Exhale and feel your abdominals engage and then lift one knee into a ninety-degree angle. Exhale again to bring up the other knee to create a tabletop with your shins. Make sure that your knees are directly over your hip bones. Pretend you're holding a tray of hot coffee on your shins.

Inhale slowly and exhale, engaging your abdominals more with each exhale. Do not release your abdominal engagement on your inhale.

Ideally, you'll hold this for thirty to sixty seconds. If you're unable to hold this position for that long at first, no problem; you can build up to it.

Attention! If this position pisses off your back, you have two options.

Adjust your knees: bring your knees a little closer toward you, which will flatten your back and eliminate any arching. If your back is still saying, "Hell, no!" stop and come out of the position cautiously by slowly bringing each foot back down to the mat, one at a time.

Side note: You may also place a small Pilates ball (nine-inch diameter) between your knees to activate your pelvic floor and abdominals. This may make the exercise feel easier.

Pilates Crawling: A Back, Pelvic Floor, and Abdominal Strengthener

This exercise has a few different options for the level of difficulty. Start slow and build up to each step. You should feel your abdominals working in each position.

Start on your hands and knees, similar to a yoga table-top position. Position your hands directly below each shoulder and your knees directly below each hip. Separate your knees hip distance apart and make sure that your low back is flat.

Lift up out of your shoulders; don't dump your weight into them. Pull in your belly button toward your spine, and close your rib cage.

Now, exhale and extend one leg out straight behind you. Hold it for three full breaths. Slowly bring it down to the starting position. Extend the opposite leg and hold for three breaths. Continue and switch to lifting one arm at a time.

Exhale and extend an arm straight out in front of you. Be sure to keep your shoulders from lifting, keep your ribs closed, and pull your navel in. Inhale and exhale three times.

Bring that arm down and switch to the next.

When you are feeling stronger, take this exercise up a notch and add two limbs.

Start by extending a leg first like you did in step 1, exhale again, and extend the opposite arm. Looking like a pointing bird dog now, you'll hold this position for three to six full breaths. Remember to keep your abs engaged and lifted, your shoulders down, and your ribs closed.

Then do this on the other side with your opposite arm and leg.

You can do this four to six times, alternating sides.

Finally, sit back into child's pose for a feel-good, back-relieving stretch (if your knees allow it).

CHAKRA
ASSESSMENTS

E ACH CHAKRA connects to physical parts of our body and relates to a specific emotion. For example, your root chakra connects to your pelvis, and its energy can impact your physical body, such as when you experience incontinence. It can also show up as a feeling, such as when you feel insecure. Assess your chakras and get curious about how they can help you increase your physical and emotional health.

Root Chakra

Problems with your root chakra can manifest as emotional issues. To find out how healthy your root chakra is, ask these questions:

- Do you tend to feel anxious in the morning when you wake up?
- Do you tend to be more frazzled than calm in general?
- Do you feel out of place?
- Has the flow of income slowed or shifted?
- Have you lost your passion or drive for things you once enjoyed?

BREATHING-PLUS-KEGELS

How do you get the energy flowing through your root chakra? Using your breath is a great start. A simple exhale engages the base of your pelvis and your pelvic floor. Adding a Kegel contraction increases the engagement. Start inhaling gently and then slowly exhaling. As you near the end of your exhale, add your Kegel contraction. Think of it as an elevator lifting from the base of your spine upward.

Sacral Chakra

Look at the list of qualities in chapter eight for the sacral chakra. As you read them one at a time, take a moment to think deeply about them. Think about who you were before kids, before pregnancy.

- Can you pinpoint when things shifted?
- How have they shifted?
- What habits have you created due to these shifts?
- How can you recalibrate life so that it feels "normal"?
- What would that take? What would that look like? Even better, what would that feel like?

Solar Plexus Chakra

Take notes of any physical symptoms that you've been feeling. Then ask yourself these questions:

Your symptoms
are not a trophy.

- Have I lost a sense of purpose?

- Have I lost my self-confidence?

- Am I standing in my power on a regular basis?

- Do I feel like I'm simply existing?

- Have I put my personal wants and needs on the back burner?

After spending some time thinking about and writing down your answers, begin answering them with ways you can create small shifts and changes to your answers.

- What would give you a sense of purpose now?

- What do you really want and need?

- What goals have you forgotten about that you'd like to pick up again? Example goals here include: Do you want to get back to a writing project? Start painting again? Did you once enjoy playing an instrument? Do you want to write a book?

Now set some specific dates for those goals. For example, some of my previous goals included getting back to dancing and performing onstage again. I did that on my fortieth birthday. Another one of those goals was getting this book written. It's been in my head for nine years, and now it is finally here! My latest goal is to become a naturopathic doctor, and I'm on the road to completing preliminary classes so that I can apply for the program.

Mark those dates in your calendar and start working on them. In no time, you'll start to feel more alive and motivated.

SOLAR PLEXUS BREATHING PRACTICE

A deep breathing practice helps calm your nervous system, optimizing brain function and giving you clarity and focus.

You can do this exercise either standing up or lying down.

Start by placing your hands over your solar plexus.

Then begin taking a deep diaphragmatic breath by taking a slow inhale for four counts, holding for two, and exhaling for five counts.

As you do this, feel your belly fill up with air and expand. Then exhale and let it relax. Repeat this five to ten times or until you feel relaxed but rejuvenated.

The Upper Chakras

Here are some questions that you can either sit with or use as writing prompts to help you assess how your upper chakra energy is functioning.

HEART CHAKRA

- Who can I be more forgiving toward?
- How can I express my empathy and compassion more?
- Who's pissed me off lately? Can I send them love anyway?

THROAT CHAKRA

- Does my throat feel tight or tickle?
- Have I expressed my needs and wants lately?

- Who do I need to share those needs and wants with?
- How can I express myself effectively?

THIRD-EYE CHAKRA

- Do you have any thoughts or visions as daydreams or night dreams?
- Have you ever thought of someone and then they happen to call or text you at that moment?

CROWN CHAKRA

- Do I feel a divine connection?
- What practice can I incorporate to feel this divine connection more?
- Do I check in with this guidance before making decisions?

Grounding Meditation

As simple as it sounds, you can use meditation and visualization to reignite energy flow through your chakras. I have a guided meditation that I use with my clients. The meditation audio recording is available at nataliesayswtf.com/wtf-book.

EMOTIONAL VIBRATION ASSESSMENT

REMEMBER THE image of the cone of vibration I shared with you in chapter eleven? The first time I saw this image and learned that our emotions vibrate at different frequency levels, it kind of blew me away. It made so much sense. Take a look at the image again and notice if you're feeling any of these emotions. Then look at the frequency number.

OMEGA

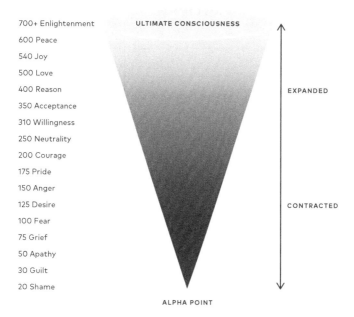

700+ Enlightenment
600 Peace
540 Joy
500 Love
400 Reason
350 Acceptance
310 Willingness
250 Neutrality
200 Courage
175 Pride
150 Anger
125 Desire
100 Fear
75 Grief
50 Apathy
30 Guilt
20 Shame

ULTIMATE CONSCIOUSNESS

EXPANDED

CONTRACTED

ALPHA POINT

For this exercise, you're going to list any emotions that you're currently feeling and then write out anything that comes to mind about these emotions.

Starting at the bottom of the cone and making your way up, take a gentle assessment of the energetic frequency levels that you're feeling right now. Are you high-vibing or could you use a frequency boost?

Jot down any of the words listed on the cone that are showing up in your life currently and then write about what may be causing this feeling. This can be a challenging exercise, so I don't recommend doing it all at once. Start slow.

When you identify what feelings resonate, write them down here. If needed, journal about them further. The idea is to see if there's any truth in these feelings and if you can release them so that you can raise your vibe, baby!

_____

_____

_____

_____

_____

_____

_____

_____

_____

_____

FINAL THOUGHTS

CONGRATULATIONS, FRIEND, you've made your way to the end of the book. I hope that it means that you've read through the exercises and created a plan of action for yourself.

I know it can feel like a lot to take on, but remember, you don't have to go vulva-to-the-wall. Pick one step and start there. You have more power than you think to feel strong, whole, and vibrant again.

It's tempting to wait for the "right" time to focus on yourself. Maybe when work slows down, or when life gets less crazy. But the truth is, there's no better time to start than right now. Your well-being doesn't need to wait. It can't. When you take care of yourself, you're better able to handle everything life throws your way—you'll be stronger, clearer, and more energized.

This isn't about perfection. It's about small, meaningful steps that put you back in touch with your body. Whether it's getting more rest, moving in ways that feel good, or finally addressing those symptoms that have been nagging you, start today. Don't wait for tomorrow or the next phase of life to prioritize yourself. You deserve to feel your f*cking best, not just someday, but now.

Your health is your foundation. Without it, you can't fully show up for your family, your work, or even yourself. And let's be real, you deserve more than just getting by. You deserve to thrive. You've made it this far, through everything life has thrown at you, and now it's time to go after those big dreams that have been put on the back burner.

Remember, you're not alone in this. There are so many women walking the same path reclaiming their health. If you need help finding a community, reach out to me and I'll find one for you! Let this be the start of your next chapter, sister. The world's waiting and the next generation depends on it.

ACKNOWLEDGMENTS

To NIA, KAIA, AND AVA, my sweet nuggets: From the days of pregnancy and bed rest to watching you grow into young adulthood, you've been my greatest teachers. Thank you for showing me all that I needed to learn so that I could share this wisdom with other mamas.

My parents, Mary and Clifford, the best grandparents who ever lived. Thank you for always being our safety net.

Gillian, thank you for reigniting my creativity, encouraging me to continue with this project, and for the introduction to Page Two.

Page Two: Jesse, Gretchen, Caela, Beate, Natassja, Sarah, Merlina, Alison, Taysia, Fiona, Michelle, Viktoria, and Madelaine. Thank you for your endless support and patience while I navigated going back to school in the middle of writing this book, and for helping me get to the finish line.

Lora and Dr. Natalie, thank you for being great friends and employers and for supporting me on my Pilates journey.

Nicole, Lindsay, and Melissa, thank you for years of friendship and support.

Dr. Cassie, Jenny Dull, Dr. Todd, Dr. Marquis, Dr. B., Harmony House Yoga, thank you for keeping me sane.

To all the moms in my community who've come through my studio and who I've met online, thank you for sharing your stories and reminding me why this book is so needed.

NOTES AND SOURCES

B ELOW YOU'LL FIND the sources I referenced throughout the book. I also highly recommend two books that were invaluable in my research: Caroline Myss's *Anatomy of the Spirit: The Seven Stages of Power and Healing* and Dr. Oscar Serrallach's *The Postnatal Depletion Cure: A Complete Guide to Rebuilding Your Health & Reclaiming Your Energy for Mothers of Newborns, Toddlers, and Young Children.*

2: It's All About the Abs

p. 38   *the history of this movement practice:* "About Pilates," Pilates Foundation, accessed October 12, 2023, https://www.pilates foundation.com/about-pilates/.

3: A C-Section Is a Major F*cking Surgery

p. 43   *the baby was removed to save the patriarchal lineage:* Allison Yarrow, "Why Are So Many Babies Born Via C-Section?" *Literary Hub*, July 19, 2023, lithub.com/why-are-so-many-babies-born-via-c-section.

p. 45   *17.4 out of 100,000 live births resulted in maternal mortality:*
"First Data Released on Maternal Mortality in Over a Decade,"
National Center for Health Statistics, Centers for Disease
Control, January 30, 2020, cdc.gov/nchs/pressroom/nchs_
press_releases/2020/202001_MMR.htm.

p. 45   *Black women in the United States are more than twice as
likely to die:* "First Data Released on Maternal Mortality in
Over a Decade."

p. 45   *After her C-section, she nearly bled to death:* Steve Gardner,
"Serena Williams Describes Near-Death Experience She Had
After Giving Birth to Daughter Olympia," *USA Today*, April 7,
2022, usatoday.com/story/sports/tennis/2022/04/07/serena-
williams-near-death-childbirth-complications/9504616002/.

p. 50   *surgeons have changed their approach to C-sections:* Linda Ha,
"C-Section Awareness Month: What Does the Surgical Procedure
Look Like?" Loma Linda University Health, April 21, 2023,
news.llu.edu/health-wellness/c-section-awareness-month-
what-does-surgical-procedure-look-like.

4: WTF Is a Pelvic Floor, and Why Is It So Important?

p. 59   *Half of adult women experience urinary incontinence:* Tarek
Khalife and Gokhan Anil, "Is Urine Incontinence Normal
for Women?" Mayo Clinic Health System, November 7, 2022,
mayoclinichealthsystem.org/hometown-health/speaking-
of-health/is-urine-incontinence-normal-for-women.

p. 64   *Kegel exercises for pelvic floor muscle strengthening:* Yi-Chen
Huang and Ke-Vin Chang, "Kegel Exercises," StatPearls, last
updated May 1, 2023, ncbi.nlm.nih.gov/books/NBK555898/.

5: WTF Is a Diastasis Recti?

p. 79   *"In 10 sessions you will feel the difference:* Joseph Pilates quoted
in Ella Riley-Adams, "How Pilates Changed My Feelings About
Fitness," *Vogue*, January 7, 2020, vogue.com/article/how-pilates-
changed-my-feelings-about-fitness.

6: WTF Is an Energetic Body?

p. 92   *there are five layers to the body:* Caroline Myss, *Anatomy of the Spirit: The Seven Stages of Power and Healing* (New York: Harmony, 1996).

p. 93   *called this energy system the biofield:* Beverly Rubik et al., "Biofield Science and Healing: History, Terminology, and Concepts," *Global Advances in Health and Medicine* 4 (November 2015): 8–14, doi.org/10.7453/gahmj.2015.038.suppl.

7: Ground and Calm the F*ck Down

p. 99   *up to 50 percent of moms may face postnatal depletion:* "Postnatal Depletion—Even 10 Years Later," goop, reviewed by Dr. Oscar Serrallach, last updated October 24, 2022, goop.com/wellness/health/postnatal-depletion-even-10-years-later/.

11: Everything Is Connected

p. 134   *"You are an emotional body:* Laura Bond, "The Emotional Body: A Method for Physical Self-Regulation," Emotional Body, accessed March 24, 2023, emotionalbody.co/resources/6/.

p. 140   *has shared his incredible healing story on many podcasts:* "A Spinal Recovery Story: Overcoming the Impossible | Dr. Joe Dispenza," *The LOAF Podcast* (Oxford University), YouTube, January 3, 2024, youtube.com/watch?v=1UXdZpQcUms.

ABOUT
THE AUTHOR

NATALIE GARAY is f*cking tired of hearing about women not receiving the resources they need to properly care for their minds and bodies after having kids, no matter how long ago it was. To help ease their pain, she has created The Natalie Garay Methode, a holistic practice specializing in pelvic floor, C-section, and diastasis recti rehabilitation.

The Natalie Garay Methode combines the physical and energetic tools that Natalie developed to heal herself from the inside out after having three daughters. These proven practices have allowed Natalie to help women of all body types, ranging from the athlete to the prenatal mama. She supports these women in her Pilates studio online and through her digital programs. Prior to opening

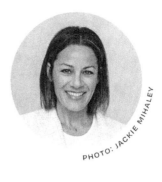

PHOTO: JACKIE MIHALEY

her own Pilates studio, Natalie worked in physical therapy clinics where she provided postoperative care. She also specializes in mindfulness practices and education about energetics to give her clients a complete mind-body-soul experience.

Natalie is also the founder and CEO of You Need {ther·happy}, the makers of therapeutic mists featuring homeopathic flower essences and organic essential oils. Their most popular product is Calm the F*ck Down. She holds a Bachelor of Arts in dance from the University of California, Santa Barbara, is a master certified Pilates instructor, a master flower essence therapist, and is on her way to becoming a naturopathic doctor.

ARE YOU F*CKING READY TO REGAIN YOUR VITALITY?

Here are a few simple ways you can kick-start your transformation.

- Follow me on Instagram for inspo at **@nataliesayswtf**

- Visit my website at **nataliesayswtf.com**

- Access additional resources, PDF downloads, and more information to help you on your healing journey at **nataliesayswtf.com/wtf-book**

- Listen to the *WTF Happened to My Body?* podcast at **nataliesayswtf.com/podcast**

- Reach out to work with me at **nataliesayswtf.com/work-with-me**

Made in the USA
Las Vegas, NV
08 March 2025

19242236R00132

SH*T YOU NEED TO KNOW AFTER HAVING KIDS

HEY, FRIEND! Have your lingering physical symptoms ever been dismissed? The message moms get is that there's nothing you can do about the aftermath of having kids, let alone the emotional roller coaster and energy-suck these symptoms cause: you just have to live with it.

WTF? *It's not f*cking true,* says rehab expert and Pilates instructor Natalie Garay: Kegels are not the be-all and end-all, peeing your pants doesn't have to be a life sentence, you don't need to have surgery to fix everything, your pain is real—and you absolutely don't just have to live with it! It's never too late to rehabilitate your body, find your sanity, and regain your vitality.

In this book, Garay shares her proven, innovative tools for regaining your physical and emotional strength. Discover what's causing your symptoms, learn the exercises that strengthen your core and pelvic floor, and find ways to increase your energy, so you can get off the roller coaster, and get back to living your life.

nataliesayswtf.com

ISBN 978-1-77458-542-9

PAGE TWO
pagetwo.com

Cover design: Taysia Louie

$17.95 USD
$21.95 CDN

9 781774 585429